W9-BUO-921

ADVANCED ELECTROCARDIOGRAPHY

Stanley T. Anderson, MB
Department of Cardiology
Alfred Hospital
Prahran, Victoria, Australia 3181

Robert L. Burr, MSEE, PhD
University of Washington
Health Science Building
Nursing Research Office
Seattle, Washington 98195

W. Gregory Downs, BSE
Research Biomedical Engineer
Division of Cardiology
University Hospitals of Cleveland
Cleveland, Ohio 44106

Carol Jacobson, RN
Cardiovascular Clinical Specialist
Swedish Hospital Medical Center
Seattle, Washington 98104

Paul Lander, PhD
Assistant Professor of Medicine
The University of Oklahoma
Health Sciences Center
Oklahoma City, Oklahoma 73104

G. Ali Massumi, MD
Adult Cardiology
Texas Heart Institute
Houston, Texas 77030

David M. Mirvis, MD
Professor of Medicine
University of Tennessee
The Health Sciences Center
Memphis, Tennessee 38163

James C. Perry, MD
Associate in Pediatric Cardiology
Texas Children's Hospital
Houston, Texas 77030

Carlos Rizo-Patron, MD
Adult Cardiology
Texas Heart Institute
Houston, Texas 77030

Published by SpaceLabs, Inc., Redmond, Washington, U.S.A.

Printed in the United States

ISBN 0-9627449-4-8

TABLE OF CONTENTS

Page

INTRODUCTION 1

1.0 LEAD SYSTEMS 3
by Stanley T. Anderson, MB

1.1 *Standard 12-Lead Electrocardiogram* 3
    1.1.1 Additional Leads 3
    1.1.2 Lead Problems 7
    1.1.3 Lead Presentation 7

1.2 *Vectorcardiography* 11

1.3 *Polar Cardiography* 11

1.4 *Monitoring* 13
    1.4.1 Bedside 13
    1.4.2 Exercise Testing 13
    1.4.3 Holter Monitoring 15
        1.4.3.1 Continuous Monitoring 15
        1.4.3.2 Intermittent Monitoring 15

1.5 *Body Surface Mapping* 15

1.6 *Magnetocardiography* 17

1.7 *Signal-Averaged Electrocardiography* 17

1.8 *12-Lead Electrocardiogram Reconstruction* 17

1.9 *Vectorcardiogram Reconstruction* 19

**2.0 CARDIAC RHYTHM
INTERPRETATION** 21
by Carol Jacobson, RN

2.1 *Interpretation of Cardiac Rhythm Strips* 21

2.2 *Rhythms Originating in the Sinus Node* 23
    2.2.1 Normal Sinus Rhythm 23
    2.2.2 Sinus Bradycardia 24
    2.2.3 Sinus Tachycardia 24
    2.2.4 Sinus Arrhythmia 25
    2.2.5 Sinus Arrest 25

2.3 *Arrhythmias Originating in the Atria* 26
    2.3.1 Premature Atrial Complex 26
    2.3.2 Wandering Atrial Pacemaker 27
    2.3.3 Multifocal Atrial Tachycardia 28
    2.3.4 Atrial Tachycardia and Paroxysmal
           Atrial Tachycardia 29
    2.3.5 Atrial Flutter 29
    2.3.6 Atrial Fibrillation 30

2.4 *Arrhythmias Originating in the AV Junction* 31
    2.4.1 Premature Junctional Complex 31
    2.4.2 Junctional Rhythm 32

Page

2.5 *Supraventricular Tachycardia* 33

2.6 *Arrhythmias Originating in the Ventricles* 33
    2.6.1 Premature Ventricular Complex 33
    2.6.2 Ventricular Tachycardia 34
    2.6.3 Ventricular Fibrillation 35
    2.6.4 Accelerated Ventricular Rhythm 35
    2.6.5 Ventricular Asystole 36

2.7 *AV Blocks* 37
    2.7.1 First-Degree AV Block 37
    2.7.2 Second-Degree AV Block 37
        2.7.2.1 Mobitz Type I Second-Degree
                AV Block (Wenckebach) 37
        2.7.2.2 Mobitz Type II Second-Degree
                AV Block 38
    2.7.3 High Grade AV Block 39
    2.7.4 Third-Degree AV Block 40

**3.0 ARRHYTHMIA DETECTION
ALGORITHMS** 41
by W. Gregory Downs, BSE

3.1 *Typical Applications of Arrhythmia
Detection Algorithms* 42
    3.1.1 Dedicated Arrhythmia
           Monitoring System 42
    3.1.2 Holter Monitoring 42
    3.1.3 Other Electrocardiographic Monitors 43
    3.1.4 Automatic Implantable Cardioverter-
           Defibrillator 43

3.2 *Signal Processing* 43
    3.2.1 Noise Sources 43
        3.2.1.1 Power Line Interference
                (60 Hz or 50 Hz) 43
        3.2.1.2 Muscle Artifact 44
        3.2.1.3 Electrode Contact Noise 44
        3.2.1.4 Baseline Wander 44
        3.2.1.5 Noise From a Single Electrode .. 45
    3.2.2 Noise Removal 45
    3.2.3 Noise Detection 45
        3.2.3.1 Primary Issues in Noise
                Detection/Rejection 47
    3.2.4 Sample Rate 47
    3.2.5 Transformations 47
    3.2.6 Beat Detection 51
    3.2.7 Feature Extraction 51
        3.2.7.1 Time Domain Features 51
        3.2.7.2 Frequency Domain Features 51
    3.2.8 Beat Classification 51
        3.2.8.1 Template Match (Correlation)
                Algorithms 51

TABLE OF CONTENTS

Page

3.2.8.2 Feature Extraction (Cluster Analysis) Algorithms 53
3.2.8.3 Hybrid Algorithms 53
3.2.8.4 Rhythm Analysis 53
3.2.9 Pacemaker Spike Detection 55
3.2.10 Ventricular Fibrillation 55
3.2.11 Lead Selection 55

3.3 Algorithm Verification 57

3.4 Current Trends in Arrhythmia Monitoring 57
3.4.1 Multiple Leads 57
3.4.2 Improved Noise Rejection 59
3.4.3 ST Segment Monitoring 59
3.4.4 Incorporation of Other Parameters 59
3.4.5 P Wave Detection 59

4.0 ST SEGMENT ANALYSIS 61
by David M. Mirvis, MD

4.1 Normal ST Segment and T Wave 61

4.2 Basic Effects of Myocardial Ischemia 61
4.2.1 Hemodynamic Consequences of Coronary Obstruction 63
4.2.2 Electrophysiologic Effects of Myocardial Ischemia 63
4.2.3 Injury Currents 63

4.3 Electrocardiographic Effects of Myocardial Ischemia 64
4.3.1 DC-Coupled Amplifiers 64
4.3.2 AC-Coupled Amplifier 64

4.4 Recording Electrocardiographic Effects of Myocardial Ischemia 65
4.4.1 ECG Lead Systems 65
4.4.2 Amplifier and Monitor Systems 67
4.4.3 Analysis Systems 67

4.5 Electrocardiographic Features of Transient Ischemia 68

4.6 Clinical Significance of Transient ST Segment Depression 68

5.0 PEDIATRIC ELECTROCARDIOGRAPHY 69
by James C. Perry, MD

5.1 Heart Rate 69

5.2 Intervals and Leads 71

5.3 Cardiac Malposition 71

5.4 Effects of Congenital Heart Defects 73

5.5 Pediatric Arrhythmias 75
5.5.1 Fetal Arrhythmias 75
5.5.2 Chaotic Atrial Tachycardia 75
5.5.3 Bradycardia in the Newborn 79
5.5.4 Developmental Aspects of Wolff-Parkinson-White Syndrome and Supraventricular Tachycardia 81
5.5.5 Junctional Ectopic Tachycardia 81
5.5.6 Permanent Junctional Reciprocating Tachycardia 81
5.5.7 Ventricular Tachycardia 83
5.5.8 Permanent Pacing Systems in Children ..83

5.6 Pediatric Electrophysiology Studies 85

6.0 HEART RATE VARIABILITY 86
by Robert L. Burr, MSEE, PhD

6.1 Physiologic Models for Heart Rate Variability Analysis 89

6.2 Heart Rate Definition Problems 89

6.3 Which to Use: Heart Rate or Heart Period? 92

6.4 Time-Weighting Versus Beat-Weighting of Statistical Summaries 95

6.5 Heart Rate Variability Measures 96
6.5.1 Kleiger Global Standard Deviation 96
6.5.2 Magid Statistic 96
6.5.3 SDANN 97
6.5.4 Ewing BB50, pNNSD, RMSSD 97
6.5.5 Frequency Versus Beatquency 99
6.5.6 Traditional Versus Autoregressive Model-Based Spectral Analysis 101

6.6 Identification of Nonsinus Beats 106

6.7 Heart Rate Variability as a Measure in Clinical Environment 109

7.0 LATE POTENTIALS AND THE ELECTROCARDIOGRAM 111
by Paul Lander, PhD

7.1 Recording the High-Resolution Electrocardiogram 111
7.1.1 Registration 113
7.1.2 Amplification and Filtering 113
7.1.3 Sampling 113
7.1.4 Isolation 115

7.2 Signal Averaging 115
7.2.1 Triggering 117
7.2.2 Signal Averaging Techniques 118
7.2.3 Noise Monitoring 119

TABLE OF CONTENTS

Page

7.3   *Time Domain Analysis of the High-Resolution Electrocardiogram* 121
     7.3.1   Filtering 123
     7.3.2   Vector Magnitude Transform 127
     7.3.3   Automatic Measurements 127

7.4   *Interpretation of Late Potentials* 129

7.5   *Frequency Domain Analysis of the High-Resolution Electrocardiogram* 129
     7.5.1   Techniques 133
     7.5.2   Spectrotemporal Mapping 133

8.0   ELECTROPHYSIOLOGY 134
by G. Ali Massumi, MD
and Carlos Rizo-Patron, MD

8.1   *Electrophysiology Equipment Requirements* 135
     8.1.1   Recording Devices 135
     8.1.2   Stimulator for Cardiac Pacing 135

8.2   *Surface Electrograms* 137

8.3   *Intracavitary Electrograms* 137

Page

8.4   *Programmed Stimulation* 137

8.5   *Cardiac Mapping* 139

8.6   *Radiofrequency Catheter Ablation* 141

8.7   *Transesophageal Pacing and Recording* 141

8.8   *Cardioversion* 143

8.9   *Defibrillation* 143

8.10   *Implantable Cardioverter-Defibrillator* 143

9.0   ABBREVIATIONS 147

10.0   REFERENCES 149

11.0   ILLUSTRATION CREDITS 155

12.0   BIBLIOGRAPHY 156

13.0   GLOSSARY 162

INDEX 166

INTRODUCTION

In the last 20 years, we have seen remarkable innovations in the diagnosis and treatment of cardiac disorders. Many of these result from the continued development of medical diagnostic instrumentation, particularly the improved interpretation and analysis the electrocardiograms. This book focuses on the enhancements of the electrocardiogram and its recording systems and the computer-based applications that have been developed over the past two decades.

Section 1.0 reviews the fundamentals of the standard 12-lead electrocardiogram and leads for specific applications. Vectorcardiography, exercise testing, and assorted monitoring techniques are also discussed.

Section 2.0 provides an overview of the electrical physiology of the heart and a guide to the interpretation of rhythm from electrocardiographic monitors.

Section 3.0 focuses on algorithms for arrhythmia detection and how their rapid advancement in real-time monitoring applies to current medical trends. Arrhythmia detection has become easier for the clinician, but increased use of these systems requires an understanding of how signal processing, noise removal, and beat detection relate to the patient's condition.

Another specialized medical application of the electrocardiogram is ST segment analysis. Section 4.0 discusses various aspects of ST segment analysis, including the effects of myocardial ischemia, coronary blockage, and transient ischemia.

Pediatric electrocardiography requires special considerations by the clinician and the biomedical equipment technician. Adult criteria do not apply to newborns, infants, or youngsters. Section 5.0 describes the particular exceptions and parameters that must be understood when assessing pediatric patients' heart rate as well as cardiac anomalies, defects, and other problems. Biplane fluoroscopy, an essential correlate of pediatric electrophysiologic studies, is also reviewed.

Heart rate variability has become a major noninvasive monitoring parameter for the influence of the nervous system on the human heart. Section 6.0 summarizes the physiologic models for heart rate variability studies and the mathematical considerations that apply to its use in patient monitoring.

Section 7.0 emphasizes how late potentials relate to the high resolution electrocardiogram, a product of advances in computer technology. The mathematical variables and theoretical concepts that led to this application are presented.

Section 8.0 describes the achievements of research and application studies in electrophysiology as they apply to the clinical monitoring of the human heart. This section reviews the current used for electrophysiology equipment as well as the interpretations of the resulting electrograms.

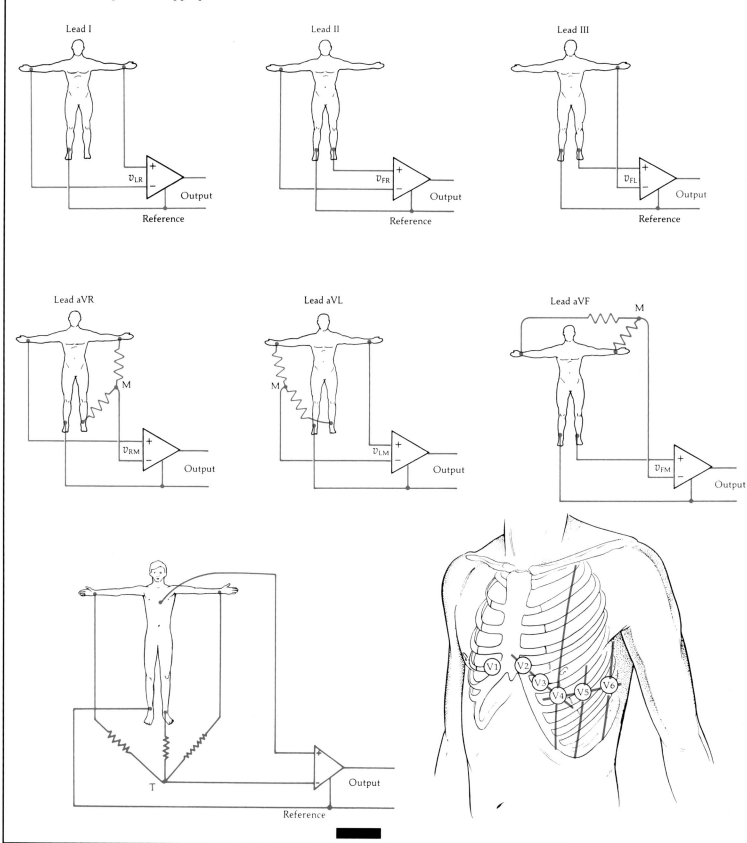

Figure 1.1–Sites of placement of standard electro-cardiographic leads for recording 12-lead electro-cardiogram with appropriate connections.

1.0   LEAD SYSTEMS

An electrocardiographic lead is a pair of polar terminals connected to electrodes. The heart approximates a double dipole layer, and the time-varying electrical field produced propagates to the surface of the body.

To reach the recording electrodes on the surface, the electrical field must pass through various tissues. This results in differing intensity of signals produced at equidistant points from the cardiac source. The display of electrical activity recorded, therefore, depends on the site of electrode placement and the lead configuration.

1.1   *Standard 12-Lead Electrocardiogram*

The reference electrode is attached to the right leg. Leads I, II, and III are bipolar leads introduced by Einthoven.[1] The augmented limb leads aVR, aVL, and aVF were introduced by Goldberger, who found that, by removing the exploring electrode from Wilson's central terminal, the amplitude increased on these "unipolar" limb leads.[2,3] The precordial leads, V_1-V_6, are "unipolar" with the electrode position on the torso following the convention of the American Heart Association.[4] A detailed discussion of leads is in an earlier publication in the Biophysical Measurement series entitled *Electrocardiography* by Charles A. Rawlings.[5] Figure 1.1 shows site placement of standard electrocardiographic leads.

The bipolar and the augmented limb leads approximate the frontal plane, while the precordial leads approximate components of the horizontal plane (Figure 1.2). Thus, the standard 12-lead recording largely describes the cardiac electrical forces in only two of the three orthogonal planes. Einthoven's rule outlines the mathematical relationship on the bipolar leads, and the relationship of the augmented limb leads is easily calculated.[1] From any two of the six standard leads, the remaining four can be derived. Similar extrapolation of the precordial leads can be made using any two as a subset. The ability to derive leads from a lessor number has been used in the computer storage and analysis of electrocardiogram (ECG) data. The clinician, however, requires information from all 12 leads for clinical diagnosis and therapeutic management.

1.1.1   Additional Leads

Other leads also provide specific clinically significant information. However, they have not been incorporated into current ECG recorders.

The Unipolar Precordial Lead: Lead V_3R, recorded with the exploring electrode in the position for V_3 but only on the right side, and V_4R aid the diagnosis of right ventricular infarction (Figure 1.3).[6] Mirror image precordial placement is required in dextrocardia. Thus, in this situation, V_1R is recorded in the same position as V_2, V_2R as V_1, and the remainder in positions as V_3 to V_6 only on the right side of the chest. To facilitate assessment, the polarity of lead I is reversed by changing the right and left arm electrodes. This results in the appropriate transposition of leads II and III and of leads aVR and aVF (Figure 1.3).

Leads V_7, V_8, and V_9 are recorded in the same horizontal line as V_4 to V_6 at the posterior axillary line (V_7), the angle of the scapula (V_8), and over the spine (V_9). These leads may be useful in the diagnosis of posterior infarction (Figure 1.4).

Figure 1.2–Orientation of the electrical axis of the standard 12 leads in relationship to the body surface.

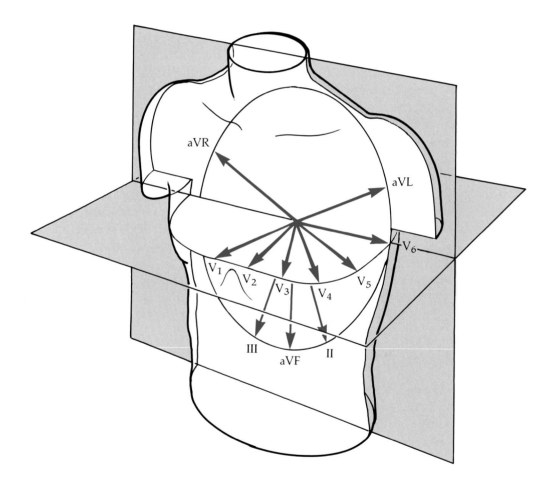

Figure 1.3–Right-sided precordial electrode sites for recording right-sided unipolar recordings.

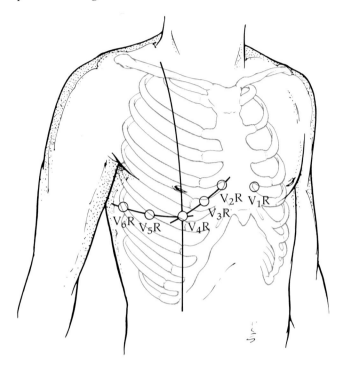

Figure 1.4–Electrode positions for unipolar leads V_7, V_8 and V_9.

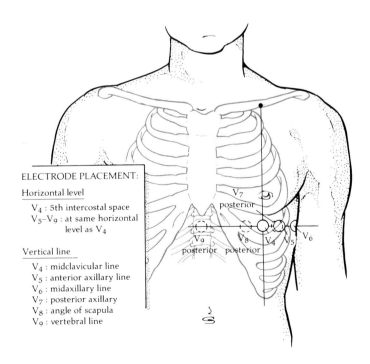

ELECTRODE PLACEMENT:

Horizontal level

V_4 : 5th intercostal space
V_5-V_9 : at same horizontal level as V_4

Vertical line

V_4 : midclavicular line
V_5 : anterior axillary line
V_6 : midaxillary line
V_7 : posterior axillary
V_8 : angle of scapula
V_9 : vertebral line

Figure 1.5–Bipolar precordial electrode sites with connections. Used for recording an "atrial" lead.

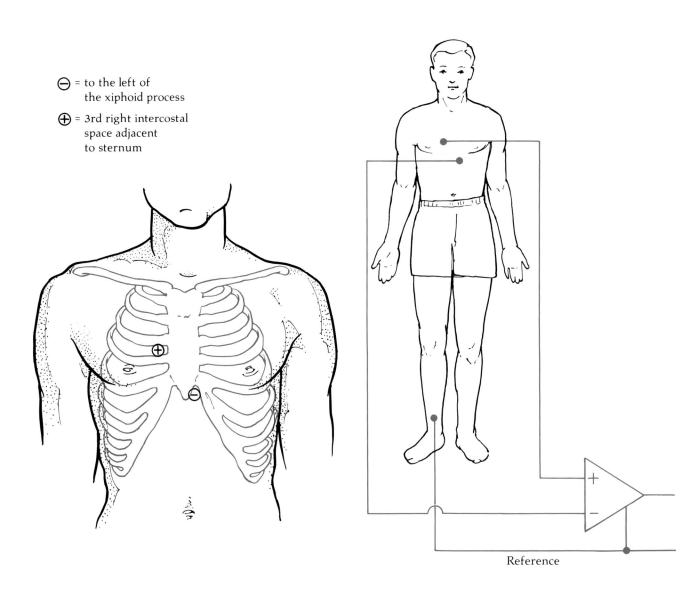

$\ominus$ = to the left of the xiphoid process

$\oplus$ = 3rd right intercostal space adjacent to sternum

Reference

Occasionally, clinicians may wish to record in other lead positions, such as one interspace higher. No accepted nomenclature exists to describe these leads. Therefore, careful annotation should be made to avoid confusion, especially when serial tracings are compared.

The Bipolar Precordial Lead: A lead, sometimes called the atrial lead, is recorded from the right of the sternum in the third interspace to the xiphoid process of the sternum to aid detection of atrial activity. Usually used for monitoring, an atrial lead can provide additional information in the differentiation of rhythm disturbances when combined with the standard ECG (Figure 1.5).

In Europe, the Nehb leads are occasionally used to access atrial activity. This presentation consists of three bipolar leads with the placement of the electrodes on the second rib at the junction with the sternum, the posterior axillary line at the level of the apex of the scapula, and on the left front of the chest at the level of the scapular apex.[7]

The Semi-Orthogonal Lead: The X, Y, and Z leads are available on some three-channel recorders and will be discussed later.

Other Leads: In the diagnosis of broad complex tachyarrhythmias, the use of unipolar or bipolar esophageal recordings in association with standard leads facilitates identification of separate atrial and ventricular activity (Figure 1.6). Post cardiac surgery epicardial electrodes are often placed to assess pacing in the postoperative period. These electrodes can record either unipolar atrial or ventricular electrograms, or can combine this information into a bipolar electrogram.

1.1.2 Lead Problems

Misplacement of electrodes is the most commonly recognized problem associated with the limb leads. Reversal of the arm leads causes inversion of lead I, with reversal of II and III, and reversal of leads aVR and aVL. The components of lead II or III may be reversed, or all three leads may be rotated clockwise or counterclockwise producing specific patterns that are important to recognize to avoid false interpretations.[8] Mispositioning of the exploring chest electrode high on the precordium or the reversal of leads can make interpretation difficult, particularly when serial comparisons are necessary.

The electrodes may be placed on any part of the arms or the left leg as long as they are below the shoulders in the former and below the inguinal fold anteriorly and the gluteal fold posteriorly in the latter.[9] When it is not possible to place the electrodes accordingly, such as with an amputation or severe burns, another more proximal placement should be used.

1.1.3 Lead Presentation

The standard 12-lead presentation commonly uses limb leads in the order I, II, III, aVR, aVL, aVF, and the precordial leads V_1 through to V_6. This is done either by grouping the leads into subsets of three displayed horizontally or in groups of six displayed vertically. Fumagalli introduced the concept of presenting aVR as — aVR and a more logical sequencing of the standard leads.[10] This presentation, subsequently popularized by Cabrera and represented in the American literature by Dower and colleagues, offers a way to use the available information more readily and turns the aVR from a relatively ignored lead into a very useful one.[11,12]

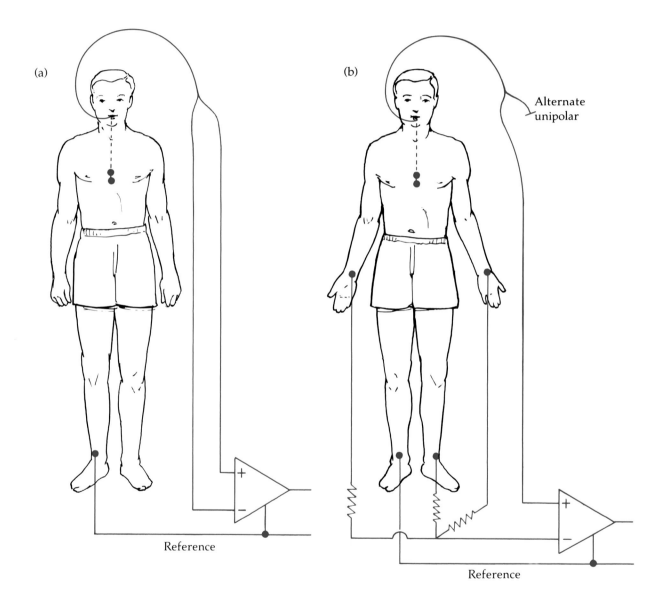

Figure 1.6–Esophageal leads. (a) Connections for bipolar recording, (b) Connections for unipolar recording (either electrode can be used).

Figure 1.7–Frank lead system and circuitry for vectorcardiography.

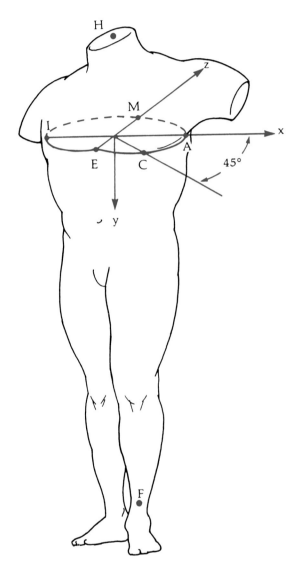

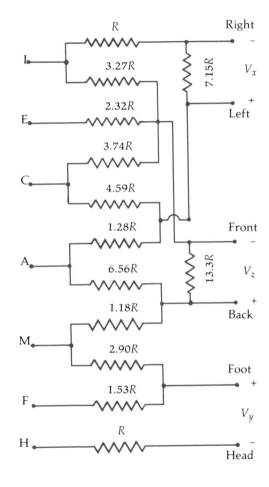

Figure 1.8–Electrode positions for the hybrid system which allows simultaneous recording of a 12-lead ECG.

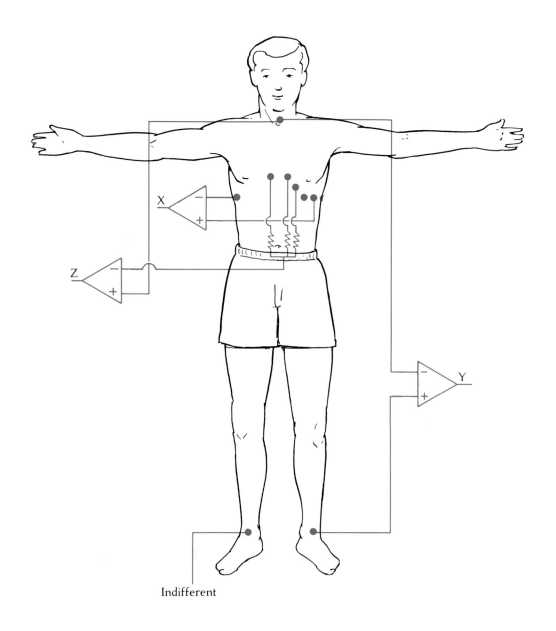

Indifferent

1.2   *Vectorcardiography*

Electrical activity radiates from the heart in all directions. Thus, a record of it in three planes that are at right angles to each other should contain more information than the standard surface recording. The recording of electrical activity in three planes requires the use of leads that represent the frontal, horizontal, and sagittal planes and is known as vectorcardiography. When the lead configuration closely approximates this situation, the leads are said to be orthogonal. For convenience of lead application (due to a reluctance to abandoning the 12-lead ECG tracing), a semiorthogonal system was developed.[16]

A semiorthogonal system includes mutual perpendicular leads in three planes by the use of the Frank lead system with the placement of the electrodes as in Figure 1.7. Resistors are placed in the circuit to correct for the magnitude of the vectors.[13] The head (H) electrode is usually positioned on the back of the neck, but can be placed on the forehead. In males, the A, C, E, I, and M electrodes are positioned in the fourth intercostal space at the left midaxillary line (A), midway between A and E (C), over the sternum (E), the right midaxillary line (I), and the spine (M). Some lead adjustment may be required in females. The level of the fifth interspace may be used to facilitate the simultaneous recording of the 12-lead ECG.

Willems and co-workers, utilizing a large series of tracings comparing the Frank leads with 12-lead recordings, concluded that "the conventional 12-lead ECG is as good as the vectorcardiogram (VCG) for the differential diagnosis of seven main entities", and "the classification results show in a quantitative way that both lead systems contain equivalent information."[14] Advantages of the VCG in comparison with the standard ECG have been well documented in selected diagnostic categories and will be considered in the discussion of the reconstructed VCG.

A less commonly used lead system was introduced by McFee and Parungao, who described it as an axial-lead system for orthogonal-lead electrocardiography.[15] A comparative study showed no significant diagnostic differences of this system when compared with the 12-lead tracing.[16]

Semiorthogonal or hybrid systems were basically designed to allow the simultaneous recording of the 12-lead ECG with X, Y, and Z leads with the latter not being true orthogonal. They add a vectorial approach to the 12-lead without the addition of many electrodes and can be readily positioned. The system, designed by Macfarlane, uses two electrodes in addition to the standard 12, has one electrode placed in the V_6R position, and the other on the back.[17] An alternative system positions the electrodes in the left and right axillas to produce lead X (Figure 1.8).[18]

1.3   *Polar Cardiography*

Polar cardiography graphically displays the magnitude and direction of the heart vector in relation to time. The lead system has not been defined. Currently, dedicated polar cardiographic recorders are no longer required since the tracing is derived, using computers, from more conventional information.

Figure 1.9–Suggested positions for routine bedside
monitoring.

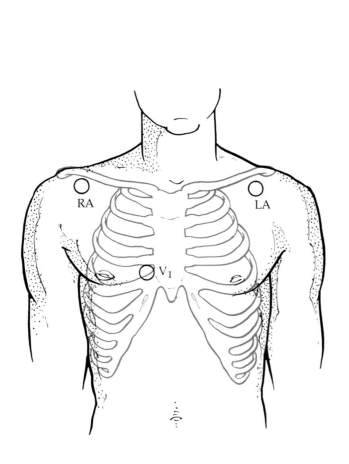

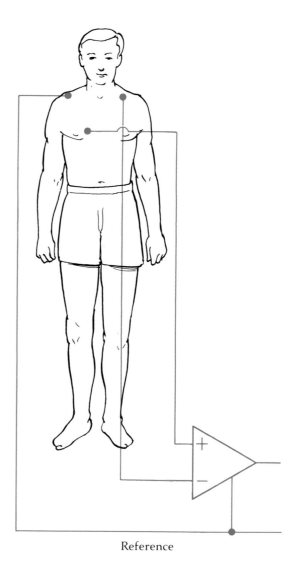

Reference

1.4   *Monitoring*

1.4.1   Bedside

Monitoring is most commonly used in patients with coronary artery disease in whom rhythm disturbances occur with a high frequency. Monitoring can be performed in a coronary care unit, an intensive care unit, an operating room, or in transit to one of these areas. The left parasternal window should remain available for the possible use of an external defibrillator and to allow easy access for clinical examination of the heart. Thus, Marriott and Fogg designed a modified bipolar lead (MCL$_1$).[19] The neutral, or ground, electrode is placed under the outer aspect of the right clavicle, the positive electrode in the position of V$_1$, and the negative electrode near the left shoulder (Figure 1.9). This configuration usually permits good visualization of atrial activity. Since alternate precordial positions are sometimes needed, bipolar leads with the positive electrode placed near the apex or on the lower left rib cage can be used.

1.4.2   Exercise Testing

Monitoring the standard 12-lead ECG usually recorded during exercise is not practical because of motion artifact introduced into the limb leads. Mason and Likar recommended moving the limb leads centrally, with little effect on the 12-lead recording.[20] They also moved the right arm electrode to the right infraclavicular fossa, medial to the deltoid insertion and 2 cm below the medial end of the clavicle, the left arm electrode to a similar position below the left clavicle, the left leg electrode midway between the costal margin and the iliac crest in the anterior axillary line, and the right leg electrode on the midthigh. Subsequently, the use of the right leg electrode positioned in the region of the right iliac fossa has become standard (Figure 1.10).[21]

Significant differences between the standard ECG and the 12 leads recorded by the above methods before and during exercise suggests that such tracing should be labelled as "torso positioned" or "nonstandard."[22] A study comparing the recommended lead positions with those of the standard 12-lead ECGs showed that inferior and posterior infarcts were lost in 69% and 31% of the recordings, respectively. Use of electrodes placed on the proximal portions of the right and left arm have produced 12-lead ECGs more closely resembling the standard tracing.[23] Subsequent investigation has shown that differences along the left arm were accentuated relative to those along the right arm and, along the left leg, an anterior site showed less deviation than did a more lateral site.[24]

Ease of placement and reduction of motion artifact has led to the popular use of bipolar precordial recordings during exercise. Usually the positive electrode is positioned at the V$_5$ level, the negative electrode being in a similar position on the right of the chest (CC5), on the manubrium (CM5), on the head (CH5), on the right arm (CR5), or the right shoulder (CS5). The CM5 position is less sensitive than the V$_5$ or the CC5 and has a more negative J point and a more positive slope.[25] When a single lead is used, then V$_5$ is the most sensitive for the detection of ischemia. However, the failure to detect ischemia with this lead alone is not specific (Figure 1.11).[26]

The use of the Frank orthogonal system has not found a significant following.[13] Thus, body surface potential mapping is experimental at present.[27]

Figure 1.10–Electrode positions for 12-lead exercise ECG as recommended by the American Heart Association.

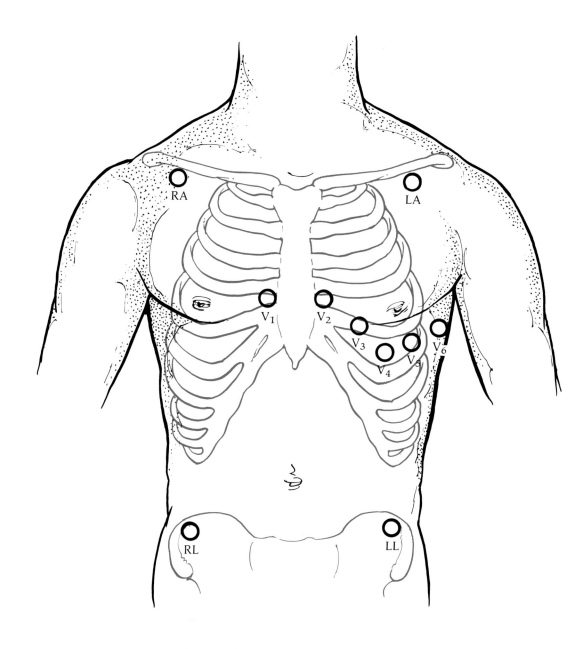

1.4.3   Holter Monitoring

1.4.3.1 Continuous Monitoring

Two-channel continuous bipolar recordings are commonly used to facilitate interpretation and to obtain some information should an electrode become detached. The American Heart Association recommends that a V_1-type lead with a positive electrode be located in the fourth right intercostal space 2.5 cm from the sternal margin, and the negative electrode over the lateral one-third of the left infraclavicular fossa.[28] Then, a V_5-type lead would accompany the positive electrode in the fifth left intercostal space at the anterior axillary line, the negative electrode being posterior 2.5 cm below the inferior angle of the right scapula. The ground electrode should be placed in the lateral one-third of the right infraclavicular fossa, but its positioning is not crucial since it is not used in the recording (Figure 1.12).

Alternative lead positioning particularly aids in the detection of ischemia by incorporating an aVF-like lead.[29,30] The generation of a third bipolar lead by alternating the recording in the second channel using a switching device has been described.[30] Use of such a system correlated with ischemic changes detected by a 12-lead exercise test. The electrodes in this system are placed between the standard V_5 position and the upper manubrium sternum to produce a bipolar V_5-like lead. A bipolar V_2-like lead is attached between the standard V_2 position and the upper manubrium sternum and an aVF-like bipolar lead is located between the ninth rib in the anterior axillary line and the upper manubrium sternum. In this system, the positive electrode is switched to a ground electrode so that the V_2 and aVF leads alternate (Figure 1.13). The use of an esophageal lead in association with a surface lead has been reported.[31]

Three-channel recorders are also available. The ground lead should be placed on the lower sternum or on the lower rib cage on the right. The positioning of the positive electrodes includes the bipolar electrodes to the left anterior axillary line (CM5), to the left midaxillary line on the lowest rib (aVF-like), and to the left sternal border at the junction of the fifth rib (CM2). The negative electrode for each lead is placed on the upper manubrium sternum (Figure 1.14).[32]

1.4.3.2 Intermittent Monitoring

The time interval between episodic "palpitations" may be such that the standard Holter recordings, even if repeated, may fail to capture significant events. Easy and quick application of electrodes is essential. This may be achieved by use of hand-held electrodes (lead I) or by the application of a small device to the chest with feet electrodes. The tracings recovered do not have a precise lead equivalent, but do diagnostically confirm the presence of and type of rhythm disturbance. The electrodes usually incorporate a mechanism for activating the recorder.

1.5   *Body Surface Mapping*

On the surface of the body, the potential field reflects the complexity of the currents and exhibits multiple maxima, minima, pseudopods, saddles, niches, and so on. These features, which convey information on the location and time sequence of the electrophysi-

Figure 1.11–Alternate sitting on the precordium for bipolar exercise ECG.

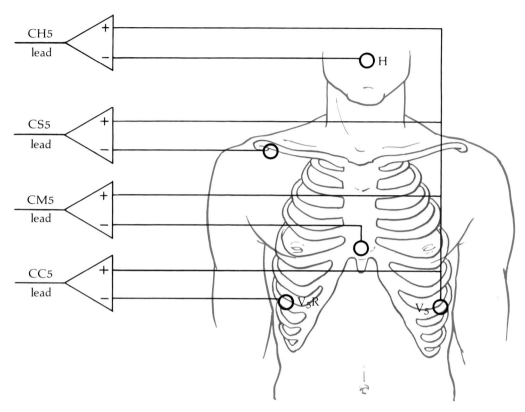

Figure 1.12–Precordial positions of electrodes for dual channel ambulatory monitoring as recommended by the American Heart Association.

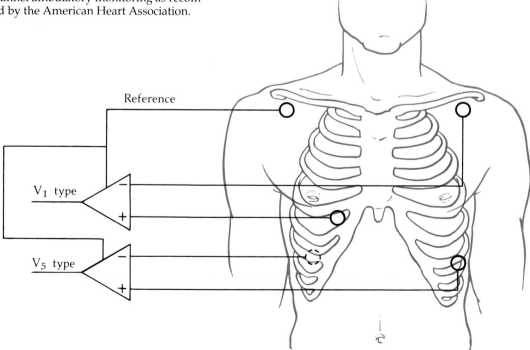

ological events of the heart, are often located in areas not explored by the 12 classical electrocardiographic leads.[33] Body surface mapping has developed as a research tool and has not been widely accepted as a clinical tool.

The number of recording sites on the chest varies from 12, i.e., 4 by 3 to 242, the distance between the electrodes being related to the number of electrodes and whether or not recording is extended on to the posterior aspect of the chest.[34,35] Since such variation in number and position exists, detailed features of each system must be selected on an individual basis. The value of continued use of this technique, as shown in a recent study, lies in the understanding gained about the relationship between pathology and the generation of the electrical signals recorded in the standard 12-lead ECG.[36]

1.6 *Magnetocardiography*

The magnetic field of the heart was first detected in 1963.[37] The magnetic signals are weak, particularly since the exploring magnet is not directly applied to the surface of the heart. The use of magnetic signals has not yet reached a clinically applicable stage.

1.7 *Signal-Averaged Electrocardiography*

The detection of ventricular late potentials using high-resolution or signal-averaged electrocardiography has had prognostic significance for the development of ventricular arrhythmias.[38] A modified or hybrid orthogonal lead system, which is as sensitive as body surface mapping, is most commonly used.[39] The standard lead configuration recommended in the time domain is an XYZ system with the X-lead electrodes placed in the fourth intercostal space in both midaxillary lines, the Y-lead electrodes on the superior aspect of the manubrium and the upper left leg or left iliac crest, and the Z-lead electrodes in the V_2 position and directly posterior from V_2 on the left side of the vertebral column (Figure 1.15).[40] Comparison with bipolar precordial leads of various types has shown a more prolonged QRS with the XYZ system and the detection of more abnormal measurements with the bipolar precordial leads.[41]

The results of high-resolution electrocardiography are lead-dependent. Accordingly, criteria and approaches established with one lead system may not be applicable to other systems. The Frank leads and modified uncorrected orthogonal leads have been used in the frequency domain. Additional studies are required to determine the optimal lead system.[40]

1.8 *12-Lead Electrocardiogram Reconstruction*

The standard 12-lead ECG remains the most commonly used for cardiac investigation because of the simplicity of the equipment required, the short amount of time needed to obtain the tracing, the amount of information recorded, and the relatively low cost of the procedure. This does not devalue other expressions of cardiac electrical activity. These offer solutions or potential solutions to signs of disturbed pathology, particularly in relation to time, such as exercise electrocardiography, Holter monitoring, or fixed monitoring. The contributions that have and will be made by the more research-orientated techniques cannot be underemphasized.

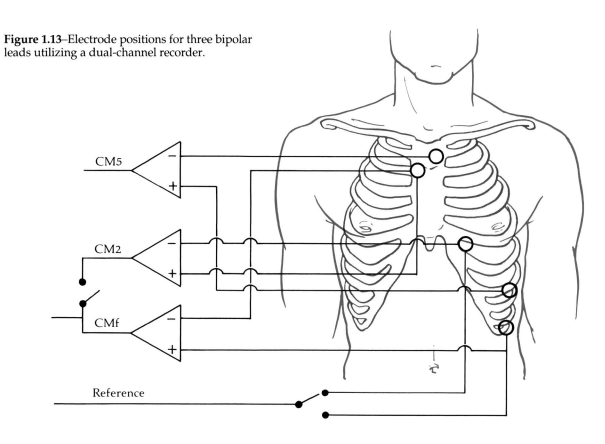

Figure 1.13–Electrode positions for three bipolar leads utilizing a dual-channel recorder.

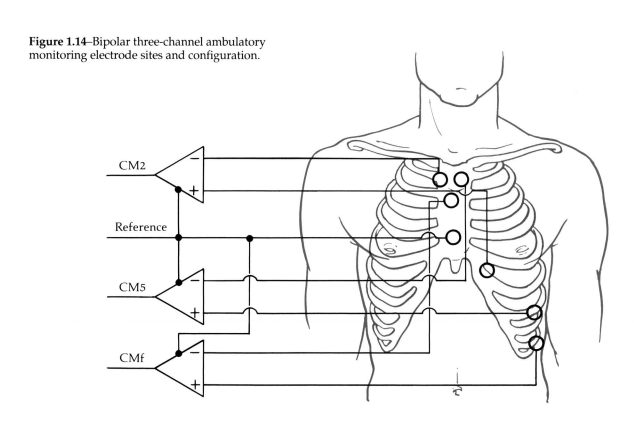

Figure 1.14–Bipolar three-channel ambulatory monitoring electrode sites and configuration.

Because of the usefulness of the standard ECG, attempts have been made to reconstruct the electrical information present in other forms of recording. The clinical applications of accurately reproducing such recordings would be of major value in exercise electrocardiography and in monitoring situations in which a potentially changing pattern of the QRS or the ST-T wave occurs over a relatively short period of time.

The electrical activity recorded at the surface depends on the geometry and resistive properties of the passive volume conductors between the source of the activity and the site of recording. Considering the anatomical position of the heart as assessed by magnetic resonance imaging, shifts of only 0.5 cm in relation to the V_2 lead have been shown to alter the reconstructed ECG, the magnitude of the error relating to the activation sequence.[42] The effect of alteration of the limb lead positions on the standard ECG has been discussed in the section on exercise testing with clear differences observed on the left arm electrode compared with the right arm electrode and with the anterior electrode compared with lateral positioning on the left leg.[24]

The problems of ECG reconstruction are of considerable magnitude. Even with slight variations occurring in the anatomical surface relationship over time, individual variations in body contour, nonuniformity of the passive volume conductors, and the recording used for derivation may not contain all the information. Reconstruction from orthogonal XYZ leads has shown minor differences between the derived tracing and the 12-lead ECG. The former correlates better with the clinical situation, and significant differences in amplitude do not influence patient treatment.[43,44]

An example of the potential value of ECG reconstruction relates to the time-dependent changes in the ST segment seen during brief coronary occlusion. This situation shows that changes determining the true magnitude and extent of the ST segment in the 12-lead ECG as conventionally recorded need to be established.[32]

1.9 *Vectorcardiogram Reconstruction*

Vectorcardiography has proved a very useful tool, particularly in the understanding of the QRS complex. Chou, in reviewing the value of vectorcardiography, indicates that it is more reliable than the ECG in the diagnosis of atrial enlargement and right ventricular hypertrophy.[44] In addition, it is more sensitive than the ECG in the diagnosis of myocardial infarction, particularly inferior myocardial infarction.[44,45] Using criteria developed in association with the ECG and recorded with a three-channel recorder so that important features of the vector QRS loop can be predicted, Warner and colleagues showed improved ability to diagnose inferior myocardial infarction.[46]

Reconstruction of the VCG from the standard 12-lead ECG, rather than recording both separately, has merit in selected cases with considerable economic savings while retaining the benefits of the information from ECG waveforms and providing additional diagnostic data. Edenbrandt and Pahlm compared three methods of VCG reconstruction and concluded that the inverse transformation matrix of Dower to be the best method of syntheses.[47] Subsequently, this method has been shown to be comparable to a regression technique.[48] The ability to derive additional information and the enhancement of electrocardiographic understanding by use of VCGs reconstructed from the standard ECG avoid the need for additional leads. Such methods could become accepted practice in selected cases if incorporated into current ECG systems.

Figure 1.15–Signal-averaged ECG electrode sites and lead configuration for time domain recordings as recommended by the task force committee of the European Society of Cardiology, the American Heart Association, and the American College of Cardiology. Note negative electrode of the Z lead is directly posterior to the V_2 position of the positive electrode.

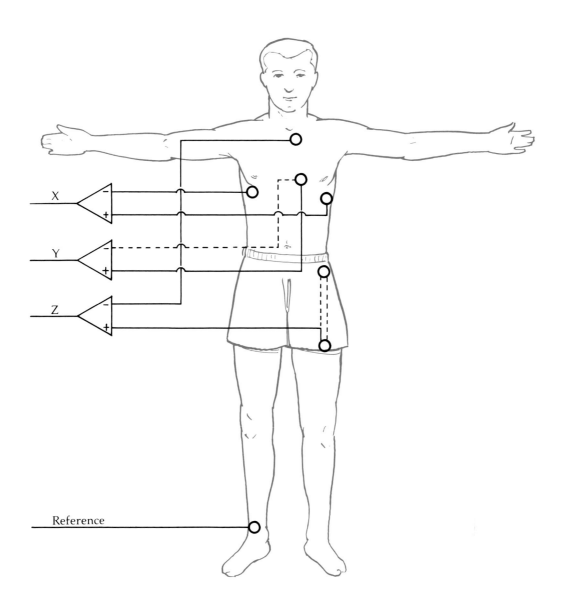

2.0 CARDIAC RHYTHM INTERPRETATION

The heart consists of two main types of cells: muscle cells and conduction cells. Atrial and ventricular muscle cells are responsible for contraction of the heart's chambers. Specialized conduction cells function to initiate and spread the electrical impulse through the heart. The electrical impulse generated in the conduction system stimulates the muscle cells to contract.

Depolarization refers to the electrical excitation of the heart resulting from the flow of ions across the membrane of cardiac cells. This wave of excitation spreads from cell to cell through the conduction system and into the muscle cells, providing the signal for them to contract.

Repolarization returns the heart to its electrical resting state, again due to ion flow across the cardiac cell membrane. Once the heart is repolarized it can again undergo depolarization.

The refractory period is the amount of time after depolarization when the heart cannot respond to another stimulus. Cardiac cells must repolarize before they can depolarize again. The refractory period occurs in two phases: (1) the absolute refractory period immediately following depolarization during which the heart cannot respond to another stimulus and (2) the relative refractory period following the absolute refractory period during which the heart can respond to a stronger than normal stimulus but with abnormally slow conduction.

Automaticity describes the ability of certain parts of the heart to initiate an impulse without an external stimulus, or spontaneously depolarize. Conductivity refers to propagation of an impulse from cell to cell within the heart. Contractility means the ability of cardiac muscle cells to shorten, or contract, in response to the electrical stimulus. Aberrant conduction refers to abnormal conduction of the impulse through the ventricles.

An arrhythmia is any cardiac rhythm that is not normal sinus rhythm at a normal rate. Arrhythmias can arise from the atria, AV node, or ventricles. Or, they can occur when conduction of the impulse from the atria to the ventricles becomes abnormal.

2.1 Interpretation of Cardiac Rhythm Strips

An electrocardiogram (ECG) is a graphic recording of the electrical activity produced by depolarization and repolarization of the heart. The ECG is recorded on standard graphic ECG paper divided into small and large boxes. The horizontal axis of ECG paper measures time and the vertical axis records voltage. The standard system uses 25 mm/sec as the dimensional unit. Each small box (1mm x 1mm) on the horizontal equals 0.04 second; one large box (consisting of five small boxes) equals 0.20 second. Vertically, each small box equals 0.1mV, one large box (five small boxes) equals 5 mV. Marks in the top margin of most ECG paper divide it into 3-second time periods.

A rhythm strip should be analyzed in an organized manner to aid in arrhythmia interpretation. The following steps are suggested:

Regularity: Determine if the rhythm is regular or irregular. This information is needed to calculate heart rate. If the rhythm appears irregular, determine if the irregularity is random or patterned (that is, repetitive groups of beats separated by pauses).

Figure 2.1—Electrographic paper showing times releative to 25 mm/sec.

R to R

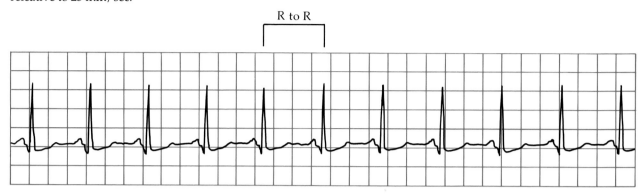

6 seconds

3 seconds

3 seconds

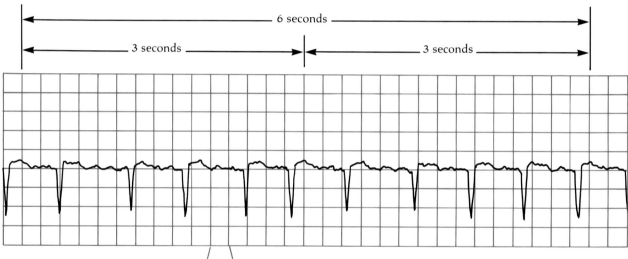

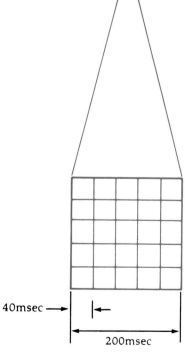

40msec

200msec

Rate: Heart rate can be obtained from the ECG strip by several methods. If the rhythm is regular, any of the following three methods can be used (Figure 2.1). Calculate atrial rate in the same way, using P waves instead of R waves:

1. Count the number of small boxes between two R waves and divide that number into 1500 (since there are 1500 small boxes in a 1-minute strip of ECG paper).

2. Count the number of large boxes between two R waves and divide that number into 300 (since there are 300 large boxes in a 1-minute strip of ECG paper).

3. If the rhythm is regular or irregular, count the number of R-R intervals in a 6-second strip and multiply that number by 10.

P Waves: Locate P waves and determine if they all look alike and if they have a consistent relationship to QRS complexes (that is, one P wave before every QRS; two or more P waves before each QRS; or random occurrence of P waves relative to QRS complexes).

PR Interval: Measure the PR interval of several complexes in a row to determine if it is of normal duration and consistent for all complexes. A normal PR interval is 0.12 to 0.20 second.

QRS Width: Measure the QRS complex and determine if it is normal or wide. A normal QRS width is 0.04 to 0.10 second.

2.2 *Rhythms Originating in the Sinus Node*

2.2.1 Normal Sinus Rhythm

The sinus node normally fires at a regular rate of 60 to 100 beats per minute (bpm). The impulse spreads from the sinus node through the atria and to the AV node, where it encounters a slight delay before it travels through the bundle of His, right and left bundle branches, and Purkinje fibers into the ventricle. Figure 2.2 presents the ECG characteristics of normal sinus rhythm:

Figure 2.2— Normal sinus rhythm.

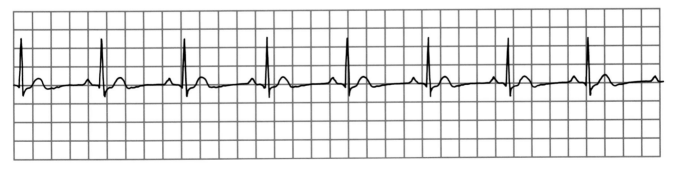

Rhythm: Regular.
Rate: 60 to 100 bpm.

P waves:	Precede every QRS complex and have a consistent shape.
PR interval:	Usually normal (0.12 to 0.20 second).
QRS complex:	Usually normal (0.04 to 0.10 second).
Conduction:	Normal through the atria, AV node, and ventricle.

2.2.2 Sinus Bradycardia

Sinus bradycardia occurs when the sinus node discharges at a rate slower than 60 bpm. The ECG characteristics of sinus bradycardia include (Figure 2.3):

Figure 2.3— Sinus bradycardia.

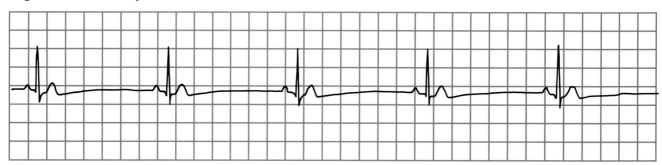

Rhythm:	Regular.
Rate:	Less than 60 bpm.
P waves:	Precede every QRS complex and are consistent in shape.
PR interval:	Usually normal (0.12 to 0.20 second).
QRS complex:	Usually normal (0.04 to 0.10 second).
Conduction:	Normal through the atria, AV node, bundle branches, and ventricles.

2.2.3 Sinus Tachycardia

Sinus tachycardia is a sinus rhythm at a rate faster than 100 bpm. The ECG characteristics of sinus tachycardia include (Figure 2.4):

Figure 2.4— Sinus tachycardia.

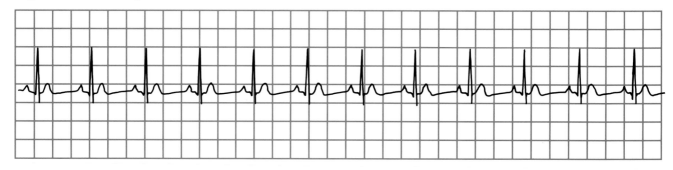

Rhythm:	Regular.
Rate:	Faster than 100 (usually 100 to 180) bpm.

P waves:	Precede every QRS complex and have a consistent shape, and may be buried in the preceding T wave.
PR interval:	Usually normal; may be difficult to measure if P waves are buried in T waves.
QRS complex:	Usually normal.
Conduction:	Normal through the atria, AV node, bundle branches, and ventricles.

2.2.4 Sinus Arrhythmia

Sinus arrhythmia occurs when the sinus node discharges irregularly. Other than a phasic increase and decrease in rate, sinus arrhythmia looks like normal sinus rhythm. The following characteristics are typical of sinus arrhythmia (Figure 2.5):

Figure 2.5— Sinus arrhythmia.

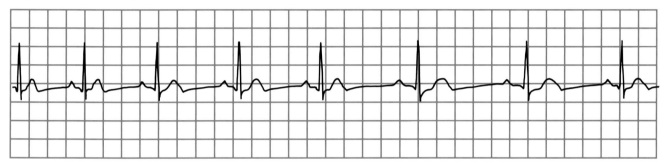

Rhythm:	Irregular; phasic increase and decrease in R-R interval (rate).
Rate:	60 to 100 bpm.
P waves:	Precede every QRS complex and have a consistent shape.
PR interval:	Usually normal.
QRS complex:	Usually normal.
Conduction:	Normal through the atria, AV node, bundle branches, and ventricles.

2.2.5 Sinus Arrest

Sinus arrest occurs when sinus node automaticity is depressed and impulses do not occur when expected. This results in the absence of a P wave at the time it should occur. The QRS complex will also be missing unless a junctional or ventricular pacemaker escapes. If only one sinus impulse fails to form, the condition is usually termed sinus pause. Sinus arrest is characterized by the following ECG changes (Figure 2.6):

Figure 2.6— Sinus arrest.

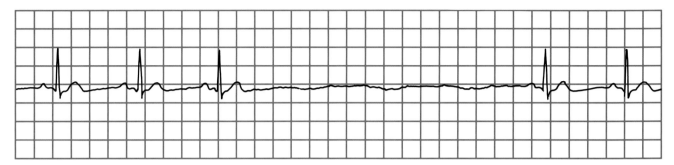

Rhythm:	Irregular due to absence of sinus node discharge.
Rate:	Atrial—usually within normal range but may fall into bradycardia range if several sinus impulses fail to form; ventricular-usually within normal range but may fall into bradycardia range if several sinus impulses fail to form and no junctional or ventricular escape beats occur.
P waves:	Present when sinus node is firing and absent during periods of sinus arrest. When present, the P waves precede every QRS complex and are consistent in shape.
PR interval:	Usually normal when P waves are present.
QRS complex:	Usually normal when sinus node is functioning and absent during periods of sinus arrest unless escape beats occur. If ventricular escape beats occur, the QRS complex is wide.
Conduction:	Normal through the atria, AV node, bundle branches, and ventricles when the sinus node fires. When the sinus node fails to form impulses, there is no conduction through the atria. If a junctional escape beat occurs, ventricular conduction is usually normal. If a ventricular escape beat occurs, conduction through the ventricles is abnormally slow.

2.3   *Arrhythmias Originating in the Atria*

Atrial arrhythmias originate in the atrial myocardium and indicate irritability in the atria. Atrial arrhythmias include premature atrial complexes (PACs), wandering atrial pacemaker (WAP), atrial tachycardia, multifocal atrial tachycardia (MAT), atrial flutter, and atrial fibrillation.

2.3.1   Premature Atrial Complex

Premature atrial beats occur when an irritable focus in the atria fires before the next sinus impulse is due. The ECG characteristics of PACs include (Figure 2.7):

Figure 2.7— Premature atrial complex (PAC).

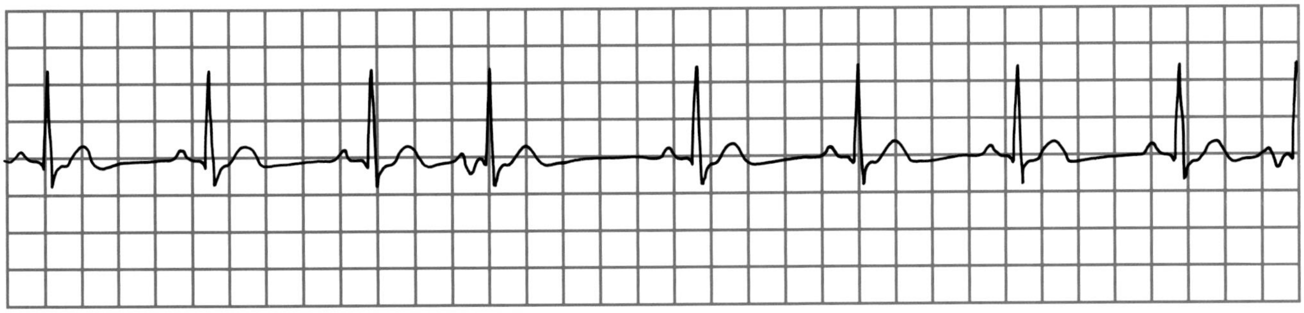

Rhythm:	Usually regular except when PACs occur, resulting in early beats.
Rate:	Usually within normal range.
P waves:	Precede every QRS complex. Configuration of the premature P wave differs from that of the sinus P waves because the premature impulse originates in a different part of the atria and depolarizes them in a different way. Very early P waves may be buried in the preceding T wave.
PR interval:	May be normal or long, depending on the prematurity of the beat. Very early PACs may conduct with a long PR interval.
QRS complex:	May be normal, aberrant (wide) or absent, depending on the prematurity of the beat. If the bundle branches have repolarized completely following the previous contraction they conduct the early impulse normally, resulting in a normal QRS. If a PAC occurs before the bundle branches have completely repolarized, the impulse may conduct aberrantly and the QRS will be wide. If the PAC occurs very early before the bundle branches or ventricles have repolarized, the impulse will not conduct to the ventricles and the QRS is absent.
Conduction:	PACs travel through the atria differently from sinus impulses because they originate from a different spot. Conduction through the AV node, bundle branches, and ventricles is usually normal unless the PAC is very early.

2.3.2 Wandering Atrial Pacemaker

WAP occurs when the site of impulse formation "wanders" from the sinus node to pacemakers in the atria or when the atria and the AV junction compete with each other for control of the heart. The morphology of P waves varies because the atria depolarize differently when they are activated from different sites. WAPs are characterized by (Figure 2.8):

Figure 2.8— Wandering atrial pacemaker.

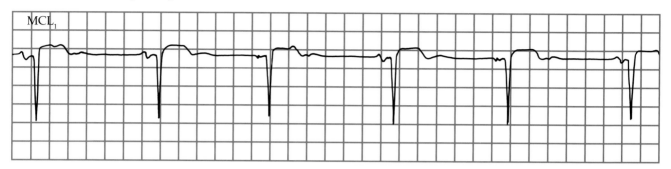

Rhythm:	May be slightly irregular.
Rate:	60 to 100 bpm.
P waves:	Exhibit varying shapes (upright, flat, inverted, notched) as impulses originate in different parts of the atrium or junction. At least three different P waves should exist to be classified as a WAP.
PR interval:	May vary depending on proximity of the pacemaker to the AV node.
QRS complex:	Usually normal.
Conduction:	Conduction through the atria varies as the atria undergo depolarization from different locations. Conduction through the bundle branches and ventricles is usually normal.

2.3.3 Multifocal Atrial Tachycardia

MAT represents the rapid firing of several ectopic atrial foci at a rate faster than 100 bpm. The ECG characteristics of MAT include (Figure 2.9):

Figure 2.9— Multifocal atrial tachycardia (MAT).

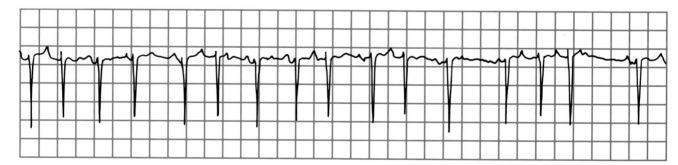

Rhythm:	Usually irregular.
Rate:	Greater than 100 bpm.
P waves:	Vary in shape because they originate in different locations in the atria. At least three different P waves must exist to be classified as MAT; usually precede each QRS complex, but some may be blocked in the AV node.
PR interval:	May vary depending on proximity of each ectopic atrial focus to the AV node.
QRS complex:	Usually normal.

Conduction: Usually normal through the AV node and ventricles. Aberrant ventricular conduction may occur if an impulse moves into the ventricles before they have repolarized completely.

2.3.4   Atrial Tachycardia and Paroxysmal Atrial Tachycardia

Atrial tachycardia is a rapid atrial rhythm occurring at a rate of 150 to 250 bpm. When the arrhythmia abruptly starts and terminates, the term "paroxysmal atrial tachycardia" is used. When the atrial rate is rapid, the AV node may begin to block some of the impulses attempting to travel through it to protect the ventricles from excessively rapid rates. This results in atrial tachycardia with AV block. The ECG characteristics of atrial tachycardia include (Figure 2.10):

Figure 2.10— Atrial tachycardia.

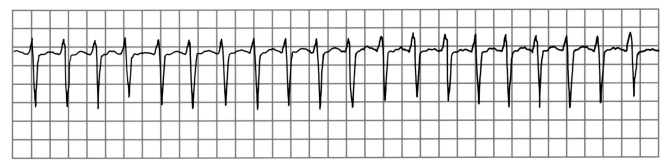

Rhythm: Regular unless variable block occurs at the AV node.
Rate: Atrial rate is 150 to 250 bpm.
P waves: Differ in configuration from sinus P waves because they originate in the atria.
PR interval: May be shorter than normal but often difficult to measure because of hidden P waves.
QRS complex: Usually normal but may be wide if aberrant conduction occurs.
Conduction: Usually normal through the AV node and into the ventricles. In atrial tachycardia with AV block some atrial impulses do not conduct to the ventricles. Aberrant ventricular conduction may occur if atrial impulses move into the ventricles before the ventricles have completely repolarized.

2.3.5   Atrial Flutter

In atrial flutter, the atria are depolarized at very rapid rates of 250 to 350 times per minutes. At such quick atrial rates, the AV node usually blocks at least half of the impulses to protect the ventricles from excessive rates. Atrial flutter most often occurs at a rate of 300 bpm, and since the AV node usually blocks half of those impulses, ventricular rates of 150 bpm are quite common. Atrial flutter is characterized by (Figure 2.11):

Figure 2.11— Atrial flutter.

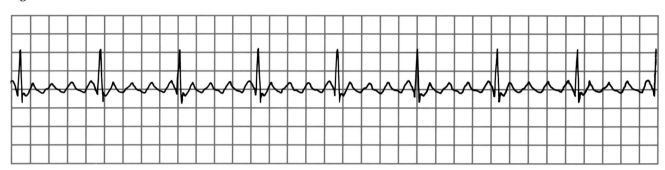

Rhythm:	Atrial rhythm is regular; ventricular rhythm may be regular or irregular due to varying AV block.
Rate:	Atrial rate is 250 to 350 bpm, most commonly 300 bpm. The ventricular rate varies depending on amount of block at the AV node, often occurs at 150 bpm with 2:1 conduction and rarely 300 bpm with 1:1 conduction. Ventricular rates can fall within the normal range when atrial flutter is treated with appropriate drugs.
P waves:	F waves (flutter waves) are seen, characterized by a very regular, "sawtooth" complex; when 2:1 conduction occurs F waves may not be readily apparent.
PR interval:	May be consistent or may vary.
QRS complex:	Usually normal; aberration can occur.
Conduction:	Variable conduction through the AV node, resulting in block of many of the atrial impulses. Conduction through the ventricles may be aberrant if impulses reach them before they have completely repolarized.

2.3.6   Atrial Fibrillation

Atrial fibrillation is an extremely rapid and disorganized pattern of depolarization in the atria, with atrial rates above 400 bpm. Atrial fibrillation is characterized by (Figure 2.12):

Figure 2.12—Atrial fibrillation.

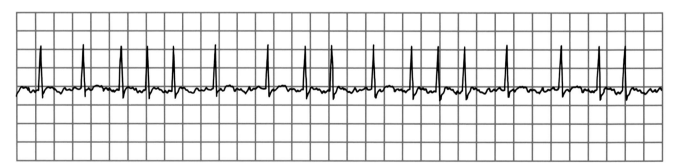

Rhythm:	Irregular; one of the distinguishing features of atrial fibrillation is the marked irregularity of the ventricular response.

Rate:	Atrial rate is 400 to 600 bpm or faster. Ventricular rate varies depending on the amount of block at the AV node. In new atrial fibrillation, the ventricular response is usually quite rapid at 160 to 200 bpm; in treated atrial fibrillation, the controlled ventricular rate occurs in the normal range of 60 to 100 bpm.
P waves:	Not present; atrial activity is chaotic with no formed atrial impulses visible. Irregular F waves often occur, varying in size from coarse to very fine.
PR interval:	Not measurable since no P waves occur.
QRS complex:	Usually normal; aberration is common.
Conduction:	Intra-atrial conduction is disorganized and very irregular. Most of the atrial impulses are blocked within the AV node; impulses conducted through the AV node usually proceed normally through the ventricles. If an atrial impulse reaches the bundle branch system before it has completely repolarized, aberrant intraventricular conduction can occur.

2.4 *Arrhythmias Originating in the AV Junction*

Cells surrounding the AV node in the AV junctional area have automaticity and can initiate impulses and control the heart's rhythm. Junctional arrhythmias include premature junctional complexes (PJC), junctional rhythms, and junctional tachycardia.

Junctional beats and junctional rhythms can appear in three ways on the ECG depending on the location of the junctional pacemaker and the speed of conduction of the impulse into the atria and ventricles.

When a junctional focus fires, the wave of depolarization spreads backward (retrograde) into the atria as well as forward (antegrade) into the ventricles. If the impulse arrives in the atria before it arrives in the ventricles, the ECG shows a P wave (usually inverted because the atria depolarize from bottom to top) immediately followed by a QRS complex as the impulse reaches the ventricles. In this case, the PR interval is very short, usually 0.10 second or less.

If the junctional impulse reaches both the atria and ventricles at the same time, only a QRS complex is seen on the ECG because the ventricles are much larger than the atria. Only ventricular depolarization is observed, even though the atria are also depolarized.

If the junctional impulse reaches the ventricles before it reaches the atria, the QRS complex precedes the P wave on the ECG. Again, the P wave usually inverts because of retrograde atrial depolarization, and the RP interval (distance from the beginning of the QRS to the beginning of the following P wave) is short.

2.4.1 **Premature Junctional Complex**

PJCs result from an irritable focus in the AV junction that fires before the next sinus impulse is due. The PJCs have the following ECG characteristics (Figure 2.13):

Figure 2.13— Premature junctional complex (PJC).

Figure 2.13— Premature junctional complex (PJC).

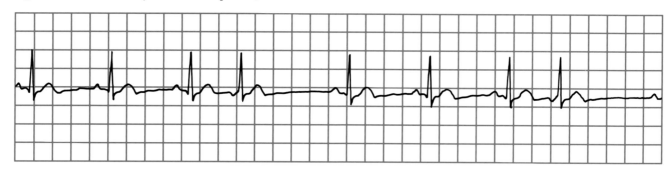

Rhythm:	Regular except for occurrence of premature beats.
Rate:	60 to 100 bpm or whatever the rate of the basic rhythm.
P waves:	May occur before, during or after the QRS complex and are usually inverted due to retrograde atrial conduction.
PR interval:	Short, usually 0.10 second or less when P waves precede the QRS complex.
QRS complex:	Usually normal, but may be aberrant if the PJC occurs very early and conducts into the ventricles during their refractory period.
Conduction:	Retrograde through the atria, and usually normal through ventricles.

2.4.2 Junctional Rhythm

Junctional rhythm can occur if the sinus node rate falls below the automatic rate of the AV junctional pacemakers. Junctional rhythms are classified according to their rate: junctional rhythm usually occurs at rates of 40 to 60 bpm, accelerated junctional rhythm occurs at rates of 60 to 100 bpm, and junctional tachycardia occurs at rates of 100 to 250 bpm. Junctional rhythm has the following ECG characteristics (Figure 2.14):

Figure 2.14— Junctional rhythm.

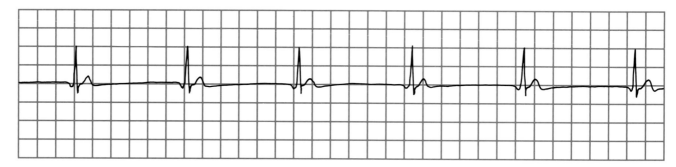

Rhythm:	Regular.
Rate:	Usually 40 to 60 bpm.
P waves:	May precede or follow QRS.
PR interval:	Short, 0.10 second or less.
QRS complex:	Usually normal.
Conduction:	Retrograde through the atria and normal through ventricles.

2.5 *Supraventricular Tachycardia*

Supraventricular tachycardia (SVT) describes narrow QRS tachycardias when the exact mechanism for the tachycardia cannot be determined from the surface ECG. SVT indicates that the rhythm originates above the bifurcation of the bundle of His (within the atria or AV junction), and that the ventricles are depolarized via the normal His-Purkinje system. Rhythms defined as SVT include sinus tachycardia, atrial tachycardia, atrial flutter, atrial fibrillation, and junctional tachycardia. Two other arrhythmias, AV nodal re-entrant tachycardia and circus movement tachycardia utilizing an accessory pathway, are also commonly considered SVT. It is important to distinguish SVT from ventricular tachycardia because this has implications for acute and long-term therapy for the arrhythmia.

2.6 *Arrhythmias Originating in the Ventricles*

Ventricular arrhythmias originate in the ventricular muscle or Purkinje system. These are considered more dangerous than other arrhythmias because of their potential to severely limit cardiac output. Ventricular arrhythmias include PVCs, accelerated ventricular rhythm, ventricular tachycardia, ventricular flutter, ventricular fibrillation, and ventricular asystole.

2.6.1 Premature Ventricular Complex

PVCs occur when an irritable focus in the ventricles fires before the next sinus impulse is due. The PVCs themselves are not harmful but may indicate increasing ventricular irritability, which can lead to more serious ventricular arrhythmias. The PVCs have the following ECG characteristics (Figure 2.15):

Figure 2.15— Premature ventricular complex (PVC).

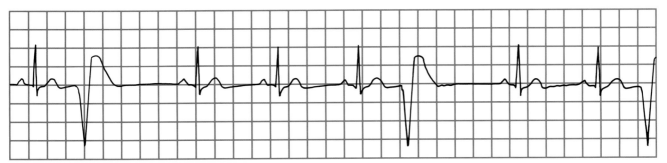

Rhythm:	Irregular because of the early beats.
Rate:	60 to 100 bpm or the rate of the basic rhythm.
P waves:	Not related to the PVCs; sinus rhythm is usually not interrupted, so sinus P waves can occur regularly throughout the rhythm. The P waves may occasionally follow PVCs due to retrograde conduction from the ventricle back through the atria; these P waves appear inverted on the ECG.
PR interval:	Not present before most PVCs. If a P wave happens by coincidence to precede a PVC, the PR interval is short.
QRS complex:	Wide and bizarre; greater than 0.10 second in duration; may vary in morphology if it originates from more than one focus in the ventricles (multifocal) and/or takes a different propagation pathway (multiform).
Conduction:	Impulses originating in the ventricles conduct through the ventricles from muscle cell to muscle cell rather than through Purkinje fibers, resulting in wide QRS complexes. Some PVCs may conduct retrograde into the atria, resulting in inverted P waves following the PVC. When the sinus rhythm is undisturbed by PVCs, the atria depolarize normally.

2.6.2   Ventricular Tachycardia

Ventricular tachycardia is defined as three or more ventricular beats in a row occurring at a rate of 100 bpm or faster. When the QRS complexes of the tachycardia are identical, the term "monomorphic ventricular tachycardia" is used. When the QRS complexes vary in shape, the term "polymorphic ventricular tachycardia" is used. The ECG characteristics of ventricular tachycardia include (Figure 2.16):

Figure 2.16— Ventricular tachycardia.

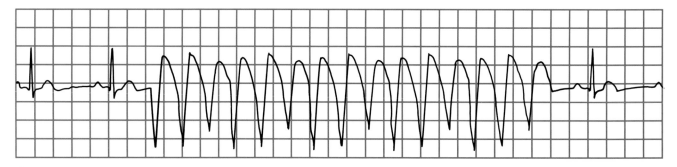

Rhythm:	Usually regular but may be slightly irregular.
Rate:	Ventricular rate is faster than 100 bpm.
P waves:	Dissociated from QRS complexes. If sinus rhythm is the underlying basic rhythm, regular P waves may occur but are not related to QRS complexes. The P waves are often buried within QRS complexes.
PR interval:	Not measurable because of dissociation of P waves from QRS complexes.
QRS complex:	Wide and bizarre; greater than 0.10 second in duration.
Conduction:	Impulses originate in one ventricle and spread via muscle cell-to-cell conduction through both ventricles. Retrograde conduction may occur

through the atria, but more often the sinus node continues to fire regularly and depolarize the atria normally. Rarely, one of these sinus impulses may conduct normally through the AV node and into the ventricle before the next ectopic ventricular impulse fires, resulting in a normal QRS complex called a "capture beat". Occasionally a "fusion beat" may occur as the ventricles depolarize via a descending sinus impulse and the ventricular ectopic impulse simultaneously, resulting in a QRS complex that appears different from both the normal beats and the ventricular beats.

2.6.3   Ventricular Fibrillation

Ventricular fibrillation refers to the rapid, ineffective quivering of the ventricles and is fatal if not immediately treated. Electrical activity originates in the ventricles and spreads in a chaotic, irregular pattern throughout both ventricles. The ECG characteristics of VF include (Figure 2.17):

Figure 2.17— Ventricular fibrillation.

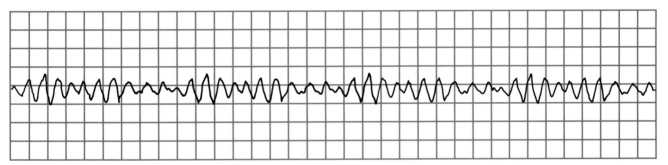

Rhythm:	Chaotic, irregular.
Rate:	Rapid, uncoordinated, ineffective.
P waves:	None seen.
PR interval:	None.
QRS complex:	No formed QRS complexes seen. Rapid, irregular undulations without any specific pattern.
Conduction:	Irregular, chaotic spread of electrical impulses through ventricles without any organized pattern.

2.6.4   Accelerated Ventricular Rhythm

Accelerated ventricular rhythm occurs when an ectopic focus in the ventricles fires at a rate of 50 to 100 bpm. The ECG characteristics of accelerated ventricular rhythm include (Figure 2.18):

Figure 2.18— Accelerated ventricular rhythm.

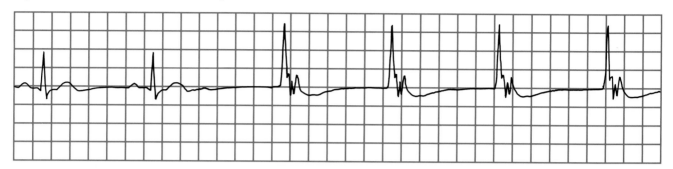

Rhythm: Usually regular.
Rate: 50 to 100 bpm.
P waves: May be seen but at a slower rate than the ventricular focus and dissoci-
               ated from the QRS complex.
PR interval: Not measured.
QRS complex: Wide and bizarre.
Conduction: If the sinus rhythm is the basic rhythm, atrial conduction remains nor-
               mal. Impulses originating in the ventricles spread via muscle cell-to-cell
               conduction, resulting in the wide QRS complex.

2.6.5   Ventricular Asystole

Ventricular asystole is the absence of any ventricular rhythm; no QRS complex, no pulse, and no cardiac output occurs. This is always fatal unless treated immediately. Ventricular asystole has the following characteristics (Figure 2.19):

Figure 2.19— Ventricular asystole.

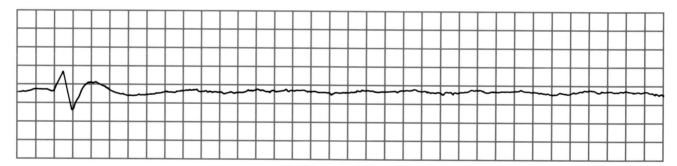

Rhythm: None.
Rate: None.
P waves: May be present if the sinus node is functioning.
PR interval: None.
QRS complex: None.
Conduction: Atrial conduction may be normal if the sinus node is functioning. No
               conduction occurs in the ventricles.

2.7   *AV Blocks*

The term "AV block" describes arrhythmias in which delayed or failed conduction of supraventricular impulses into the ventricles occurs. AV blocks are classified according to the location of the block and to the severity of the conduction abnormality.

2.7.1   First-Degree AV Block

First-degree AV block is defined as prolonged AV conduction time of supraventricular impulses into the ventricles. This delay usually occurs within the AV node, and all impulses conduct to the ventricles, but with delayed conduction times (longer PR intervals). First-degree AV block can be recognized by the following ECG characteristics (Figure 2.20):

Figure 2.20— First-degree AV block.

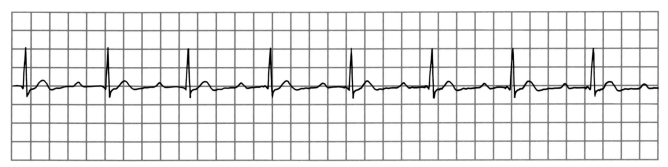

Rhythm: Regular.
Rate: Can occur at any sinus rate, usually 60 to 100 bpm.
P waves: Normal, precede every QRS complex.
PR interval: Prolonged above 0.20 second.
QRS complex: Usually normal.
Conduction: Normal through the atria, delayed through the AV node, and normal through the ventricles.

2.7.2   Second-Degree AV Block

Second-degree AV block occurs when one atrial impulse at a time fails to be conducted to the ventricles. Second-degree AV block falls into two distinct categories: Mobitz Type I block, usually occurring in the AV node, and Mobitz Type II block, occurring below the AV node in the bundle of His or the bundle branch system.

2.7.2.1   Mobitz Type I Second-Degree AV Block (Wenckebach)

Mobitz Type I second-degree AV block, often referred to as Wenckebach, is a progressive increase in conduction times of consecutive atrial impulses into the ventricles until one impulse fails to conduct, or is "dropped". This appears on the ECG as the gradual lengthening of PR intervals until one P wave fails to conduct and is not followed by a QRS complex, resulting in a pause after which the cycle repeats itself. Mobitz Type I second-degree AV block has the following ECG characteristics (Figure 2.21):

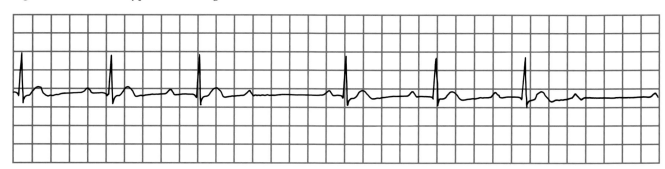

Rhythm:	Irregular; overall appearance of the rhythm demonstrates "group beating" (groups of beats separated by pauses).
Rate:	Can occur at any sinus or atrial rate.
P waves:	Normal; some P waves are not conducted to the ventricles, but only one at a time fails to conduct.
PR interval:	Gradually lengthens in consecutive beats. The PR interval preceding the pause is longer than that following the pause.
QRS complex:	Usually normal unless an associated bundle branch block occurs.
Conduction:	Normal through the atria, but progressively delayed through the AV node until an impulse fails to conduct. Ventricular conduction is normal. Conduction ratios can vary, with ratios as low as 2:1 (every other P wave is blocked) up to high ratios such as 15:1 (every 15th P wave is blocked).

2.7.2.2 Mobitz Type II Second-Degree AV Block

Mobitz Type II second-degree AV block is the sudden failure of conduction of an atrial impulse to the ventricles without progressive increases in conduction time of consecutive P waves. Mobitz Type II block occurs below the AV node and is usually associated with bundle branch block; therefore, the dropped beats are usually a manifestation of bilateral bundle branch block. This form of block appears on the ECG much the same as Mobitz Type I block except that no progressive increase in PR intervals occurs before the blocked beats. Mobitz Type II block is less common, but more serious, than Mobitz Type I block. Mobitz Type II second degree AV block has the following ECG characteristics (Figure 2.22):

Figure 2.22— Mobitz Type II second-degree AV block.

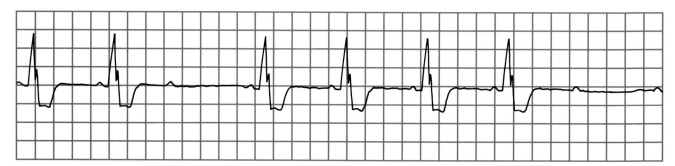

Rhythm:	Irregular due to blocked beats.
Rate:	Can occur at any basic rate.
P waves:	Usually regular and precede each QRS complex. Periodically a P wave is not followed by a QRS complex.
PR interval:	Constant before conducted beats. The PR interval preceding the pause is the same as that following the pause.
QRS complex:	Usually wide due to associated bundle branch block.
Conduction:	Normal through the atria and through the AV node but intermittently blocked in the bundle branch system, thus failing to reach the ventricles. Conduction through the ventricles is abnormally slow due to associated bundle branch block. Conduction ratios can vary from 2:1 to only occasional blocked beats.

2.7.3 High Grade AV Block

High grade AV block occurs when two or more consecutive atrial impulses are blocked when the atrial rate is less than 135 bpm. If the atrial rate is very fast, as in atrial flutter with atrial rates of 300 bpm, physiological AV block results as a normal function of the AV node and therefore cannot be called high grade block, thus the arbitrary atrial rate limit of 135 bpm. High grade AV block may be Mobitz Type I, occurring in the AV node, or Mobitz Type II, occurring below the AV node. High grade block can be recognized by these following ECG characteristics (Figure 2.23):

Figure 2.23— High grade AV block.

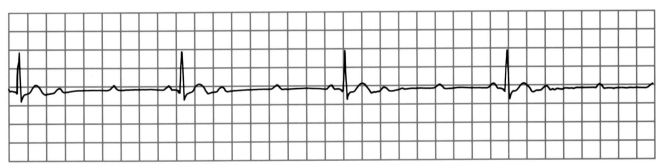

Rhythm:	Regular or irregular, depending on conduction pattern.
Rate:	Atrial rate less than 135 bpm.
P waves:	Normal, present before every conducted QRS complex, but several P waves are not followed by QRS complexes.
PR interval:	Constant before conducted beats. May be normal or prolonged.
QRS complex:	Usually normal in Mobitz Type I block and wide in Mobitz Type II block.
Conduction:	Normal through the atria; two or more consecutive atrial impulses fail to conduct to the ventricles. Ventricular conduction is normal in Mobitz Type I and abnormally slow in Type II block.

2.7.4　Third-Degree AV Block

Third-degree AV block is complete failure of conduction of all atrial impulses to the ventricles. In third-degree AV block, complete AV dissociation occurs. The atria are usually under the control of the sinus node or an atrial pacemaker and the ventricles are controlled by either a junctional or ventricular pacemaker. Third-degree AV block demonstrates the following ECG criteria (Figure 2.24):

Figure 2.24— Third-degree AV block (complete block).

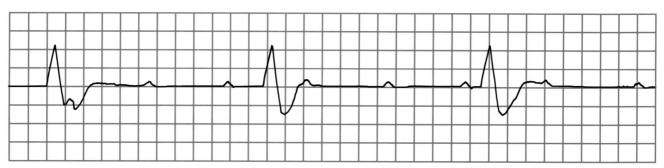

Rhythm:	Regular.
Rate:	Atrial rate is usually normal, the ventricular rate less than 45 bpm.
P waves:	Normal but dissociated from QRS complexes.
PR interval:	No consistent PR intervals because no relationship exists between the P waves and QRS complexes.
QRS complex:	Normal if ventricles controlled by a junctional pacemaker, but wide if controlled by a ventricular pacemaker.
Conduction:	Normal through the atria. All impulses are blocked at the AV node or in the bundle branches, so there is no conduction into the ventricles. Intraventricular conduction is normal if a junctional escape rhythm occurs and abnormally slow if a ventricular escape rhythm occurs.

3.0 ARRHYTHMIA DETECTION ALGORITHMS

Modern arrhythmia detection algorithms are becoming increasingly sophisticated as rapidly improving computer hardware enables them to perform more complex tasks. However, the basic process by which these algorithms function has remained fundamentally unchanged since the early days of computerized electrocardiogram (ECG) monitoring.

Computer monitoring of the ECG began in the late 1950s when a system was developed to detect P waves and QRS complexes from the ECG waveform.[49] This work was expanded through the early 1960s; in 1965, the first program to attempt analysis of the ECG based on computer-extracted measurements was introduced.[50] Improvements in computer analysis of the diagnostic 12-lead ECG continued to be made through the next decade. Today, many of these algorithms are still used in substantially unchanged forms.

In the 1970s, the emphasis of development efforts changed from the diagnostic ECG, which gathered about 1 minute of ECG information and analyzed it in extensive detail, to real-time monitoring of the ECG for detection of arrhythmias. The arrhythmia detectors developed then and those currently in wide use are essentially premature ventricular contraction (PVC) detectors because ventricular information is considerably easier than atrial information to detect and analyze and has been generally considered to be more clinically significant. The shift to real-time arrhythmia detection occurred primarily in response to the view of the medical community that life-threatening occurrences of ventricular fibrillation (VF) were frequently preceded by a high incidence of PVCs. The first commercial arrhythmia monitoring systems became available in the late 1970s. During the 1980s, arrhythmia detection algorithms grew increasingly sophisticated and commercial arrhythmia monitoring systems became commonplace.

All arrhythmia algorithms share certain common structures, although the emphasis, implementation, and form which these structures take largely depends on the setting in which the algorithm operates: ambulatory (Holter) or real-time (ICU, telemetry, and others). Figure 3.1 illustrates the basic form of an arrhythmia detection algorithm.

Figure 3.1– Flow diagram of an arrhythmia detection algorithm.

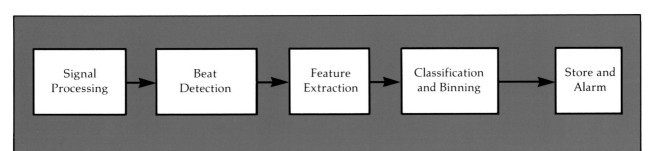

3.1 *Typical Applications of Arrhythmia Detection Algorithms*

3.1.1 Dedicated Arrhythmia Monitoring System

In its most common use, that of a dedicated arrhythmia monitor, an arrhythmia detection algorithm processes an ECG signal from a patient who is connected via a cable to a bedside monitor or wearing a telemetry transmitter. The arrhythmia monitor should detect all abnormal occurrences in the ECG and notify the clinician by means of an audible alarm, a visual alarm, and/or a hard-copy printout if any life-threatening arrhythmias occur. These arrhythmia detection algorithms commonly detect abnormal (ectopic) QRS complexes without distinguishing between ventricular and supraventricular beats, VF, runs of ventricular tachycardia (VT), runs of supraventricular tachycardia, pauses, and asystole. Monitoring ST segment activity for detection of myocardial ischemia is also becoming increasingly common. Frequently, the arrhythmia monitor forms a part of a larger integrated patient monitoring system which may also measure blood pressures (invasive and noninvasive), cardiac output, blood oxygen level, temperature, respiration, and other parameters. It is also usually connected by a computer communication network to other monitors in the same hospital unit, other areas of the hospital, or even outside the hospital, thus allowing remote access to the arrhythmia information.

An arrhythmia detection algorithm for this application must run in real-time, never fail to trigger an alarm if a life-threatening event occurs, and provide some degree of storage and user review capability.

3.1.2 Holter Monitoring

A Holter monitor is a small recording device that stores ECG waveforms for 24 or 48 hours on a magnetic cassette tape or in solid-state computer memory. This monitor is usually employed to obtain a comprehensive picture of ECG during normal daily activity. The stored information is then analyzed at high speed by a Holter scanner that can produce a full disclosure printout (a very compressed view of the entire 24 or 48-hour period), complete arrhythmia information, and ST segment information.

The off-line nature of a Holter scanner arrhythmia algorithm provides a major advantage over an algorithm in a real-time application. Questionable segments of data can be examined several times using different processing techniques. Sections of intermittent noise can be scanned both forward and backward, allowing more accurate detection of the end of a noise event and quicker return to processing. Since a user reviews all the scanner's decisions and can override any beat classification, the algorithm can be less stringent in its definition of noise. This permits the user to delete noise that the algorithm has classified as ectopy while minimizing the potential for loss of useful information. Alarms for specific arrhythmias would be meaningless in an off-line arrhythmia detection algorithm since the ECG is usually processed hours or days after it actually occurred.

Another less common type of Holter monitor is the event recorder, which contains a real-time arrhythmia detection algorithm. Only abnormal events are stored in its digital memory, therefore no full disclosure ECG is available.

3.1.3 Other Electrocardiographic Monitors

These include diagnostic 12-lead, ST segment monitoring, heart rate variability (HRV), and late potential devices. Although these devices are not arrhythmia monitors as such, abnormal beats must be detected in order to achieve accurate readings of the desired parameter since each of these tests is defined for nonectopic beats only. Typically, the ST segment, diagnostic 12-lead ECG and late potential tests employ some signal averaging in their algorithms. Any abnormal beats that are included in the signal averaging can skew the results and perhaps even obscure the parameter being measured.

3.1.4 Automatic Implantable Cardioverter-Defibrillator

With the recent advent of the automatic implantable cardioverter-defibrillator (AICD), there has been a great deal of interest in optimizing the algorithms which detect VF and VT from electrodes implanted in the myocardium. The algorithm in each AICD must detect the onset of VF or VT very accurately and very quickly in order to trigger defibrillation or cardioversion.

3.2 *Signal Processing*

The goal of signal processing as it relates to arrhythmia detection is to eliminate as much noise as possible while retaining as much of the actual ECG signal information as possible. In order to remove the noise from the signal, it is necessary to understand the characteristics of both the ECG signal and the potential forms of noise.

3.2.1 Noise Sources

3.2.1.1 Power Line Interference (60 Hz or 50 Hz)

Most monitoring systems have a notch filter that removes this very common type of interference (Figure 3.2).

Figure 3.2– (a) Power line interference (b) Removed by a notch filter.

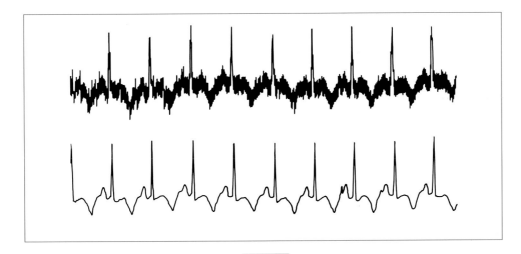

3.2.1.2 Muscle Artifact

Contraction of a muscle under an ECG electrode will cause noise to appear in the ECG signal, as shown in Figure 3.3. Unfortunately, this type of noise has a bandwidth similar to the ECG signal and, therefore, cannot be eliminated by simple filtering. Placement of the electrodes over areas with relatively little skeletal muscle can minimize the amount of muscle tremor artifact.

Figure 3.3– Noise resulting from muscle contraction.

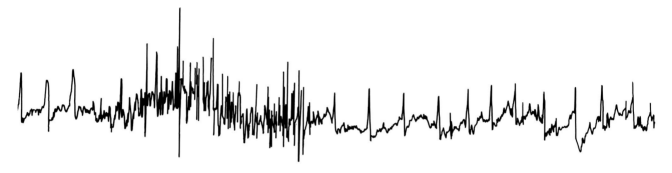

3.2.1.3 Electrode Contact Noise

Any disturbance of the electrical signal path from the body to the ECG amplifier will cause extensive pin-to-pin noise that completely obscures the actual ECG waveform. This is most often caused by an electrode in poor contact with the skin, perhaps due to poor adhesive, lack of good skin preparation, or absence of conducting gel between the electrode and the skin. Another frequent cause of electrode contact type noise is a partial break in the wire that connects the electrode to the patient ECG cable or a loose connection between this wire and the patient cable. Figure 3.4 shows typical noise resulting from poor electrode contact.

Figure 3.4– Typical noise resulting from poor electrode contact.

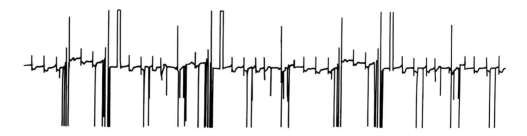

3.2.1.4 Baseline Wander

Low-frequency wander of the ECG signal can be caused by respiration or patient movement (Figure 3.5).

Figure 3.5– Low frequency wander in ECG signal.

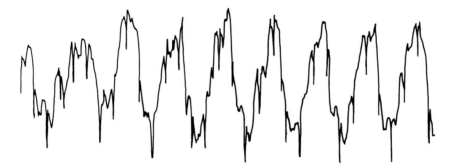

3.2.1.5 Noise From a Single Electrode

Electrode contact noise and muscle tremor usually originate from one electrode site. If the noise persists, its source can be traced to a specific electrode using the knowledge of how each lead is derived from each electrode. For example, if noise appears on leads II and III, but lead I is clean, then the noise must be originating from the left leg electrode. If noise is present in *all* leads, then it is possible that the right leg electrode is faulty since it is used by all leads as the reference ground.

3.2.2 Noise Removal

If it were necessary for arrhythmia detection algorithms to make decisions based on preset definitions of "normal" and "abnormal", as is the case in a diagnostic 12-lead ECG, then it would be necessary to analyze a bandwidth that preserves all the features of the original ECG signal (about 0.0 Hz to 500 Hz).[51] However, arrhythmia monitoring's task is to distinguish *differences* in beats from a given patient's dominant rhythm and morphology. Therefore, no real need exists to carefully preserve all of the features of the original waveform in signal processing. A rather narrow bandwidth that removes low frequency baseline wander as well as a large part of the muscle tremor noise can be used (Figure 3.6).

However, extreme overfiltering of an ECG waveform can also be counterproductive. Narrow, large amplitude noise spikes may be slurred, giving them longer duration and smoother features. This can cause a spike, that is clearly noise in the unfiltered or minimally filtered ECG, to look like an actual QRS complex when it reaches the arrhythmia algorithm (Figure 3.7).

3.2.3 Noise Detection

An arrhythmia detection algorithm should recognize when the noise content of the ECG becomes so great that it obliterates the signal content, and stop attempting to detect beats until an adequate ECG signal returns. One of the most common ways of detecting an unprocessable signal is to determine if an electrode no longer makes good contact with the skin. Contact quality can be easily determined by constantly measuring the resistance between any two electrodes. Although the resistance from a new properly applied and maintained electrode through the body to another good electrode is fairly high, it still is

Figure 3.6–Lead II with muscle tremor and baseline wander; then same segment after a bandpass filter (3 to 15 Hz).

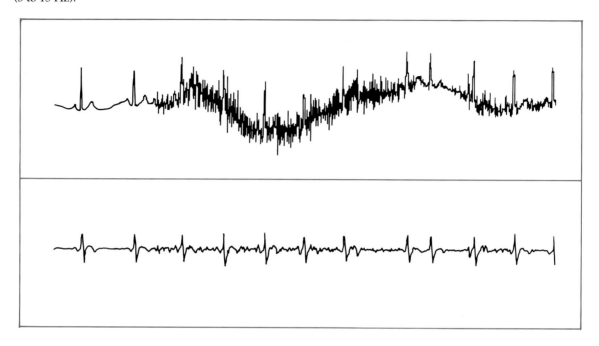

Figure 3.7–In the top tracing, the momentary spike is clearly noise, but in the lower tracing, which has been passed through a 3 to 15 Hz filter, what was obviously a dominant beat now appears to be an abnormal beat.

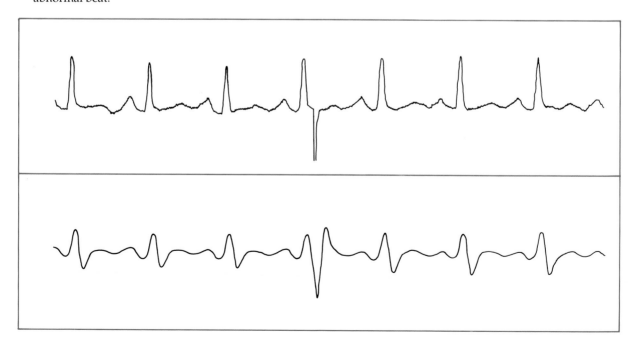

much lower than if either of the electrodes is off the body (infinite resistance), partially detached, or dried out. A continuity check to determine the quality of electrode contact is frequently performed in the preamplifier hardware, which passes the information on to the software algorithm.

The most common "noise detector" in arrhythmia detection algorithms is a simple routine that checks the unfiltered ECG for some common noise situations, such as signal saturation at either the high or low limit of the amplifier, high frequency muscle artifact indicated by a large number of crossings of the zero line, or sudden large amplitude-deflection of the baseline.

3.2.3.1 Primary Issues in Noise Detection/Rejection

The designer of an arrhythmia detection algorithm faces three major dilemmas concerning noise:

1. What is the best way to quantify/recognize noisy sections of ECG data?

2. What level of noise should the algorithm allow before it stops processing?

3. After an algorithm stops processing due to noise, how does it know when to start again?

3.2.4 Sample Rate

The sampling rate of arrhythmia detection systems ranges from a low of 100 samples per second (sps) to a high of 500 sps. Naturally, with the lower sampling rates, higher frequency events and features will be lost; but for detection of typical premature ventricular beats, higher frequency components are not required.

3.2.5 Transformations

In addition to noise removal and detection, preprocessing of the ECG signal can also take the form of an algorithm that performs some real-time analysis and transforms the data stream into another waveform that can be more easily analyzed by the beat detection and classification algorithms. A preprocessor known as Amplitude-Zone-Time-Epoch-Coding (AZTEC) was developed in the late 1960s. This algorithm compresses high sampling rate information into a series of straight line segments that can then be processed by later algorithm stages in an effectively much lower sampling rate (Figure 3.8).[52]

AZTEC was designed to minimize low-amplitude high-frequency noise and, at the same time, reduce data rate while retaining necessary information about the QRS complexes. Although this preprocessor is no longer employed in modern arrhythmia detection algorithms, it was the first widely used preprocessor and strongly influenced subsequent arrhythmia systems.

Figure 3.8–An ECG trace before (top) and after (bottom) AZTEC transformation. The period between beats, which contains little useful information, is compressed into a single straight line.

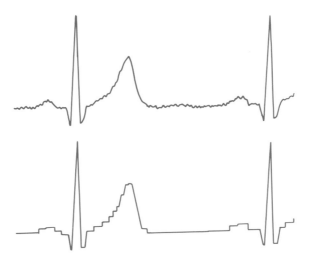

Figure 3.9–Beat is detected each time the voltage crosses a threshold, which is a fraction of the average peak amplitude.

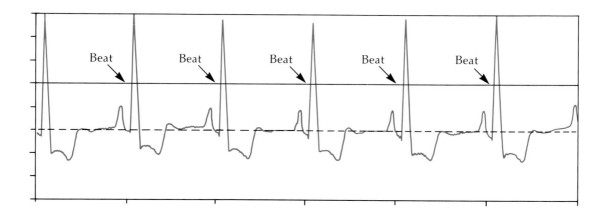

Table 3.1—Time Domain Features

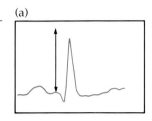
(a)

(a) Height

The height of a candidate beat is measured as the maximum-minimum voltage in the region of interest. The maximum and minimum voltages may be determined from the whole beat or from a part of the beat. In the example at right, they are measured from the entire beat.

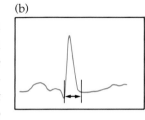
(b)

(b) Width or Duration

The width of a beat can be measured from onset to offset of the QRS complex, as in the example at right, or at a point of higher voltage, such as the beat detection threshold. This second method produces a smaller value for beat width, but is more immune to error. The terms width and duration are used interchangeably, the difference being that width is thought of as the feature measured on a strip chart printout of an ECG and duration as the actual feature being measured, independent of strip chart paper speed.

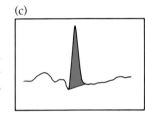
(c)

(c) Area

The calculation of area can also be performed in several different ways. The total absolute area from onset to offset may be measured as shown at right, or the measurement may be of total positive area, total negative area, the difference between positive and negative area, or area above the beat detection threshold.

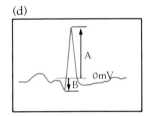
(d)

(d) DC Offset

DC offset is a calculated parameter which indicates whether a beat is primarily positive or negative. Using the beat at right, the DC offset is $(A-B)/(A+B)$. Therefore, a value of 0 indicates that the beat is evenly positive and negative, with a positive value indicating positive deflection and negative value indicating negative deflection.

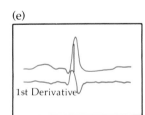
(e)

(e) Maximum and Minimum Slope

The maximum and minimum values of the first derivative can be used as separate features since they represent the maximum upslope and downslope during the QRS complex.

Polarity or Direction or Orientation

These three terms all indicate whether a beat is primarily positive or negative.

Time (premature or late)

Both the R-R interval preceding a beat and the interval following a beat can be considered features and may be used by some algorithms as such.

P-R interval

If P-wave detection is being performed, then this interval can be considered a feature.

Shape

Measurement of shape is performed in conjunction with correlation analysis. Some arrhythmia detection algorithms extract only shape. The part of the beat used for shape analysis varies from algorithm to algorithm and can include as much as the entire beat (with P and T waves), or as little as a particular portion of the QRS complex.

Figure 3.10–Three dominant beats and one PVC
with their frequency spectrums determined by FFT.

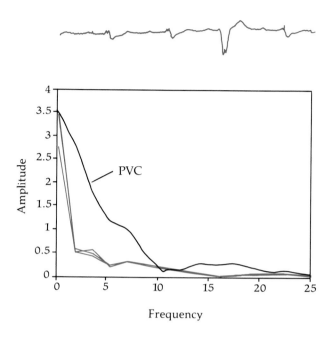

Figure 3.11–The dominant beat in the upper figure
forms a template which is clearly violated by the
PVC in the lower figure.

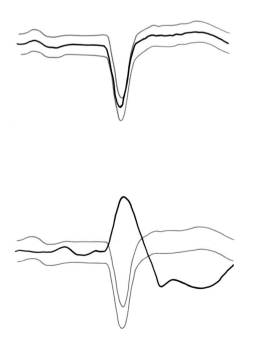

3.2.6   Beat Detection

Virtually all arrhythmia detectors detect QRS complexes by using a threshold trigger (Figure 3.9). The waveform used for detection can be a raw ECG, a filtered ECG, the output of a preprocessor, or some other derived waveform (ECG derivative, spatial magnitude of a multiple lead system, or others).[53] The threshold for triggering a beat is usually dynamic, rather than static, so that it can adjust to gradual changes in amplitude over time.

Most QRS detectors have a "no-look" period after detecting a beat during which they do not even look for potential beats. This period can be no more than the minimum possible interval between two actual QRS complexes. If a heart rate of 350 beats per minute (bpm) is considered beyond the maximum physiologically possible rate, then a "no-look" interval of 170 milliseconds is probably acceptable (0.170 second=60 seconds per minute/ 350 bpm).

3.2.7   Feature Extraction

Once a QRS complex has been found by the beat detector, it is characterized by a set of features so that it can be classified as normal or ectopic.

3.2.7.1 Time Domain Features

Some of the time domain features which may be extracted by an arrhythmia detection algorithm appear in Table 3.1.

3.2.7.2 Frequency Domain Features

A Fast-Fourier Transform (FFT) can be performed on the data segment containing the individual beat, providing an analysis of the frequency content of the beat. The spectrum for any morphology should be quite distinctive, as shown in Figure 3.10. The inclusion of an integrated circuit chip called a digital signal processor (DSP) into a system can greatly speed the execution of FFTs, easing the computational requirements on the rest of the system and making their inclusion into a real-time application much more feasible.

3.2.8   Beat Classification

Once a detected beat is divided into its set of features, an arrhythmia detection algorithm must next decide whether the beat is dominant or ectopic. If it is ectopic, then further classification may be performed. For example, ectopic beats with similar shapes may be grouped together and distinctions made between ventricular and supraventricular beats. Traditionally, arrhythmia detection algorithms have fallen into two groups: the "template match" or "correlation" algorithms, and the "feature extraction" or "clustering" algorithms.

3.2.8.1 Template Match (Correlation) Algorithms

This class of algorithms uses shape (also called morphology) to distinguish dominant from ectopic beats. The shape of the normal beat is used as a template to which new beats

Figure 3.12–Three features were extracted from the continuous strip shown above. The scatter plots show that different morphologies tend to group in feature space. The numbers in parentheses indicate how many beats are in each cluster.

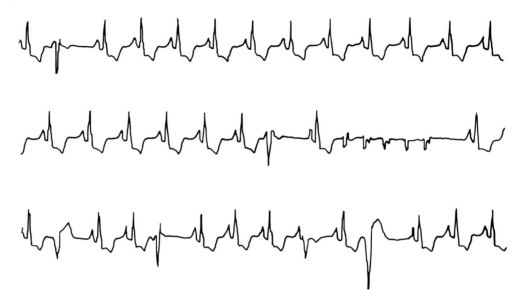

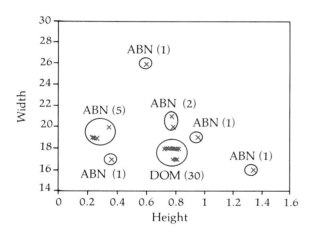

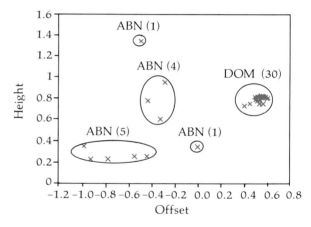

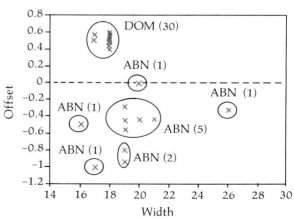

are compared. When a beat violates the dominant template, as shown in Figure 3.11, it is classified as ectopic.

The template match type of comparison has the advantage of being very intuitive, since the algorithm is performing essentially the same procedure that a human observer would use through a visual comparison of the shapes of two beats. Template matching has one disadvantage in that the correlation procedures used to distinguish differences in shape are somewhat mathematically intensive and therefore require a fast computer system to achieve real time processing. Another disadvantage relates to the implementation of the correlation calculation. To make an accurate determination of the correlation between two waveforms, they must be aligned very carefully. The algorithm must find a stable fiducial point within each beat that acts as a landmark to enable exact alignment of like-shaped beats. The simplest landmark is the maximum amplitude, but several others exist that are less sensitive to error, such as the point of maximum positive, or negative, slope.

3.2.8.2 Feature Extraction (Cluster Analysis) Algorithms

An arrhythmia detection algorithm that uses only features, as opposed to shape, can distinguish dominant from ectopic beats by finding the "clusters" in the parameter space. With only two parameters under consideration (n=2), the visual analogy is simple, as shown in Figure 3.12.

This process of looking for clusters is valid for any number of parameters, although when more than three parameters are used, the traditional graphical representation is no longer possible.

The advantages of using only feature extraction in a beat classification algorithm include relative simplicity from a computational standpoint, and a reduction in importance of subtle changes in dominant morphology which may cause a dominant beat to violate a template. The use of multiple parameters buffers the effect of any single feature.

The obvious disadvantage to using feature extraction rather than template matching is that the beat morphology is no longer an explicit part of the decision-making process. This means that the algorithm is not analogous to the method which a trained human observer would use in separating dominant and ectopic beats.

3.2.8.3 Hybrid Algorithms

A frequent compromise to the dilemma of whether to use template matching or feature extraction for classification of beats is to use a hybrid of the techniques. Generally, the template match is the most important element in deciding whether a beat is dominant or ectopic, but multiple features can be used with varying degrees of importance to assist in the final decision. This combination of the two methods of beat classification takes the advantages of each method while attempting to minimize the disadvantages.

3.2.8.4 Rhythm Analysis

In addition to morphologic information and extracted features, the timing of each beat in relation to its surrounding beats is an important factor in classifying beats as dominant or

Figure 3.13–The event between the third and fourth beats can be rejected with a high degree of confidence since it is interpolated (does not interrupt the normal rhythm) and it falls late in the interval between the two normal sinus beats.

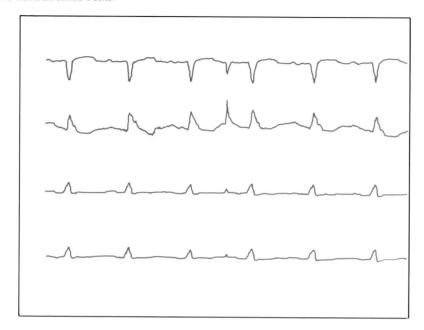

Figure 3.14–A single-lead arrhythmia monitor using lead III would determine this PVC to be a pause, since its amplitude is almost 0 in that lead. However, multiple-lead monitoring could easily determine that this is a PVC.

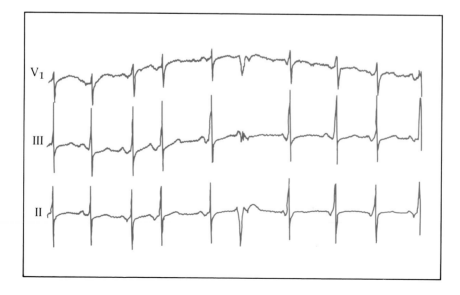

ectopic. Physiologically impossible occurrences can be ignored. For example, if two ectopic beats are detected between two on-time dominant beats, then these ectopic beats are probably isolated noise events which have passed through the front-end noise detection rather than an interpolated couplet (Figure 3.13).

Rhythm analysis also encompasses the relatively simple post-beat classification definitions of pauses (a longer than usual time between consecutive dominant beats), supraventricular tachycardia (several consecutive dominants at an accelerated rate), and VT (several consecutive ectopic beats at an accelerated rate).

3.2.9 Pacemaker Spike Detection

Detection of pacemaker spikes generally is not an issue in development of an arrhythmia detection algorithm. This task is usually performed by a special hardware circuit that analyzes the raw analog ECG signal. The digitally-sampled signal lacks the high-frequency, low-amplitude information necessary to reliably detect pacer spikes from surface electrodes. Accurate detection of pacemaker spikes by the front end is very helpful to the arrhythmia algorithm since paced beats have a distinct morphology often different from the unpaced dominant and should not be grouped with ectopic morphologies.

3.2.10 Ventricular Fibrillation

Due to their life-threatening nature, VF and VT must **always** be found by an arrhythmia detection system. To decrease the response time of a system to VF, the ECG signal is frequently passed through the VF algorithm before being sent on to the beat detector or even the signal processing section. Various techniques have been proposed over the years to detect VF, many using a combination of time domain and frequency domain information, with heavy emphasis on the latter.[54,55]

The older algorithms were developed using surface electrodes and since the ECG signal has different characteristics when viewed using implanted electrodes, new algorithms have been required. The incidence of false VF/VT alarms for AICD algorithms must be nearly 0, because any detection of VF or VT causes the defibrillator or cardioverter to discharge, resulting in pain to the patient and shorter battery life. Since batteries must be replaced by surgical procedure, this consideration is not trivial.

3.2.11 Lead Selection

Arrhythmia detection algorithms can function using any ECG lead (or combination of leads in a multiple-lead system) because discrimination of dominant and ectopic beats is independent of any absolute definitions and detection of VF is not lead-dependent. In a multiple-lead system, lead selection should attempt to provide orthogonal information to the arrhythmia monitor. Using orthogonal leads, an ectopic beat that occurs in a direction perpendicular to one of the monitored leads (resulting in very low amplitude) has higher amplitude in the other lead(s) (Figure 3.14). For this reason, the default leads in most two-lead arrhythmia monitoring systems are II and V_1.

Figure 3.15–The first row consists of the labels assigned to each beat by a theoretical arrhythmia detection algorithm. N=normal, V=ventricular ectopic beat. The ninth beat in the strip went undetected by the arrhythmia detector. The second and third rows represent how each beat label is evaluated as far as the class of dominant beats and abnormal beats.

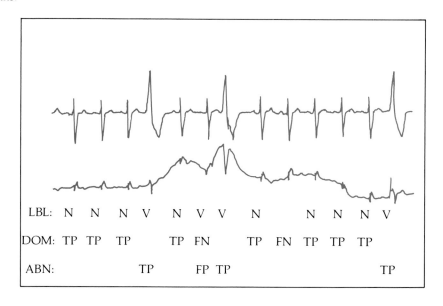

Figure 3.16–Multiple-lead monitoring enables an algorithm to continue processing on one lead while the others are noisy.

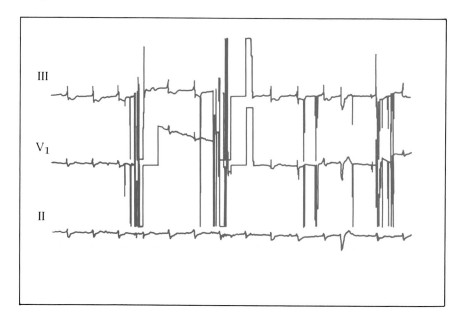

3.3 *Algorithm Verification*

Three terms commonly used in evaluation of arrhythmia detection algorithms are defined below:

True Positive (TP): An event occurred and was accurately detected.
False Negative (FN): An event occurred and was not correctly detected by the device.
False Positive (FP): No event actually occurred, but one was detected by the device.

Figure 3.15 shows a strip of ECG, some sample classifications by a hypothetical (and very poor) arrhythmia detection algorithm, and the evaluation of each event. An ideal algorithm would have 100% TP, 0% FN, and 0% FP. The impact of FNs and FPs on user confidence is very strong, especially with respect to VF and VT. If an arrhythmia monitoring system misses any occurrence of VF or VT (FN), then users may never trust that system. On the other hand, if a system frequently alarms for VF or VT when in fact none has occurred (FP), then users may ignore alarms, and perhaps even turn off the audible alarm tones.

Two large databases of annotated ECG data containing a very wide variety of arrhythmias and noise are currently available. The American Heart Association (AHA) database contains 160 separate 3.5 hour, two-channel Holter-type tapes or digital files.[56] For each file, the last 30 minutes are completely annotated with beat labels and rhythm information. One half of this database is available for general distribution to aid in development and in-house testing of arrhythmia algorithms, while the other half is kept by the Emergency Care Research Institute (ECRI) for periodic evaluations of available systems. Another database, developed at the Massachusetts Institute of Technology and Beth Israel Hospital, consists of 48 (30-minute) two-channel digital files obtained from Holter recordings.[57]

The Association for the Advancement of Medical Instrumentation (AAMI) has published a set of recommendations for testing ventricular arrhythmia detection algorithms to be used in conjunction with the standard available annotated databases.[58]

When examining any statistics of arrhythmia algorithm performance, it is crucial for the user to know whether the algorithm was developed using the same database which was used for evaluation. If this is the case (that is, retrospective rather than prospective evaluation), then the statistical data is not necessarily a true indication of how well the algorithm performs in actual use on prospective ECG data. For this reason, the ECRI evaluations of arrhythmia detection systems using the confidential half of the AHA database should be considered the best available assessment of device performance.

3.4 *Current Trends in Arrhythmia Monitoring*

3.4.1 **Multiple Leads**

Many current real-time arrhythmia monitors have now implemented algorithms which enable them to process the ECG in two leads, as has been the case for Holter monitoring for some time. Dual-lead monitoring increases the likelihood that even during periods of transient noise there will exist one processable lead (Figures 3.16 and 3.17) while decreasing the likelihood that an ectopic event will be of such low amplitude in all monitored leads that it will be missed (Figure 3.14).

Figure 3.17–Noise originating from the RA electrode would cause any arrhythmia system not monitoring lead III to incorrectly decide that this rhythm is ventricular tachycardia. This noise was caused by a respiratory therapy treatment known as "clapping".

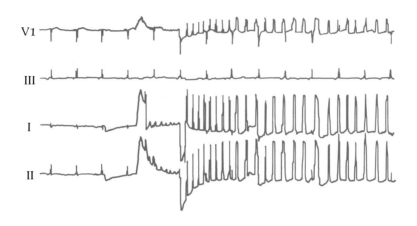

Figure 3.18–Excessive contact noise on the ECG leads completely obscures the QRS complexes, but it is obvious from the continued normal rhythm of the blood pressure pulses that a normal ECG rhythm is present under the noise.

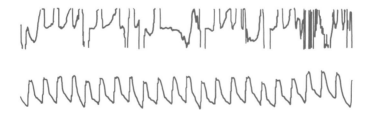

With faster, more powerful microprocessors available it is likely that arrhythmia detection algorithms will soon be able to process more than two leads, thus increasing accuracy and reducing FPs.

3.4.2   Improved Noise Rejection

Detection and classification of QRS complexes on a perfectly clean ECG signal is a relatively simple process, one performed quite adequately by most current arrhythmia monitoring systems. What truly separates the useful algorithms from the less useful ones is how they deal with a signal of less than ideal quality. Improvement of noise handling algorithms will undoubtedly be an issue in the future development of arrhythmia detection algorithms. This is true not only for dedicated arrhythmia monitoring systems, but also for arrhythmia algorithms in devices that monitor other electrocardiographic diagnostic parameters such as late potentials, heart rate variability, and ST segment levels.

3.4.3   ST Segment Monitoring

To accurately measure ST segment changes over time, all ectopic beats and all normal beats even slightly corrupted by noise must be eliminated from analysis. Any nondominant beats that are included in ST segment analysis can skew the results since the ST segment deviation for an abnormal beat is likely to be much different than that of the dominant morphology and is meaningless to any trending of myocardial ischemia.

3.4.4   Incorporation of Other Parameters

If an arterial blood pressure is being monitored concurrent with arrhythmia detection in the same patient bedside monitor, the beat onset and rhythm information present in the blood pressure waveform can aid the arrhythmia detection algorithm. One useful situation is shown in Figure 3.18, in which the ECG tracing is totally useless due to intermittent electrode contact noise. In a normal arrhythmia detection algorithm there would be no cardiac rhythm information available at all. However, analysis of the arterial pressure tracing clearly demonstrates that the heart is still beating at a normal rate.

3.4.5   P Wave Detection

Clinically, a major limitation of all current arrhythmia monitoring systems is their inability to provide any information about atrial activity due to the very small amplitude of the P wave relative to the QRS complex. The P wave is frequently obscured by even a minor level of baseline noise. No methods for reliable P wave detection from surface electrodes placed in the standard configuration have yet been developed. For an arrhythmia monitor to perform its function to the highest degree, it must detect **all** arrhythmias, ventricular (QRS complex) and supraventricular (P wave). Some early ECG monitoring algorithms attempted to detect P waves by searching backwards from a detected QRS complex for the preceding P wave.[49] With the advent of multiple lead systems, P wave detection may be somewhat more feasible since adequate P wave amplitude is more likely to be present in one of several available leads than in a single lead.

Figure 4.1–A typical cardiac action potential.

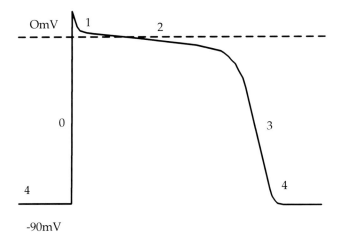

Figure 4.2–(a) Transmembrane action potentials recorded simultaneously from an endocardial and epicardial cell on the normal left ventricle. (b) Schematic representation of intracellular potentials in endocardial and epicardial cells at the moment of the vertical line in the top panel.

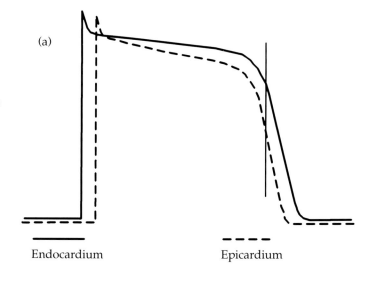

Endocardium   Epicardium

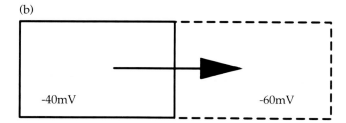

4.0   ST SEGMENT ANALYSIS

The heart normally undergoes a repetitive sequence of electrical activation (depolarization) followed by recovery (repolarization). Potentials generated by activation of the ventricles produce the QRS complex of the electrocardiogram (ECG). The ST segment and T wave reflect potentials generated by the repolarization of the cardiac ventricles. This section examines the importance of monitoring changes in ST segment produced by transient myocardial ischemia. Specific areas reviewed include the physiologic mechanisms underlying the production of the normal ST segment and T wave, the abnormalities in these processes resulting from myocardial ischemia, how these abnormalities affect the ECG, how these abnormalities can be recorded, and the clinical significance of ECG changes.

4.1   *Normal ST Segment and T Wave*

Action potentials recorded from cardiac cells have a characteristic appearance (Figure 4.1). Activity begins from a baseline level determined by the transmembrane resting potential or phase 4 potential. During this period, the inside of the cell is negative in relation to the cell exterior, having a normal transmembrane potential gradient of approximately –90 mV. Activation of the cell results in a rapid shift in intracellular potential to positive values, producing the upstroke or phase 0 of the action potential. Intracellular potentials then fall back to negative levels as the cell repolarizes or recovers. This occurs in three phases: an initial brief rapid phase (phase 1), followed by a prolonged relatively stable period (phase 2 or plateau phase), and a final period of rapidly falling potential (phase 3).

The normal ST segment is produced by differences in the duration of action potentials across the ventricular wall.[59] Normally, action potentials are shorter near the epicardial surface than near the endocardium (Figure 4.2). Thus, cells near the epicardium complete repolarization before endocardial cells.

The differences in recovery times result in potential differences between cells across the ventricular wall (Figure 4.2). Cells near the epicardium that recover more rapidly have intracellular potentials that are more negative than do cells near the endocardium that recover later. Positive currents then flow in intracellular space from more positive (less repolarized) to more negative (more repolarized) cells.

Intracellular current flow thus proceeds from endocardium to epicardium. An electrocardiographic electrode over the heart or on the body surface senses current flowing toward it and registers positive potentials. Hence, the normal ST segment is positive and the normal T wave is upright.

4.2   *Basic Effects of Myocardial Ischemia*

Myocardial ischemia results from an insufficient supply of oxygen and other nutrients to meet the metabolic demands of cardiac tissue. When flow cannot maintain the normal functions of the cell but can sustain cell life, myocardial ischemia occurs. If oxygen supply is reduced to lower levels at which cell life cannot be maintained, myocardial infarction develops.

Ischemia can result from an increase in oxygen demand in myocardial tissues, a reduction in coronary artery blood flow or, most commonly, a combination of both factors.[60] The three major determinants of oxygen demand are heart rate, myocardial contractility,

Figure 4.3–(a) Simultaneously-recorded action potentials from an epicardial and an endocardial cell in the heart with subendocardial ischemia. (b) Schematic of intracellular potentials in the two cells during phase 4 [vertical dashed line in (a)]. (c) Potentials during phase 3 [solid vertical line in (a)] are more negative in the ischemic endocardial cell than in the epicardial cell.

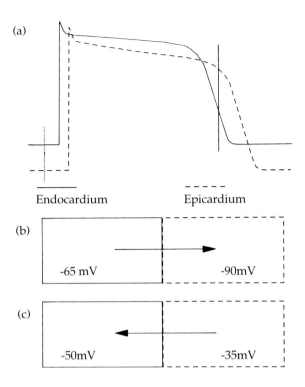

(a)

Endocardium   Epicardium

(b)

-65 mV   -90mV

(c)

-50mV   -35mV

Figure 4.4–(a) Diastolic injury current produces TQ-segment elevation in the DC coupled recording. (b) Systolic injury current produces ST-segment depression in the recording. (c) In the capacitor coupled recording, the TQ-segment elevation and ST-segment depression summate to yield only ST-segment depression.

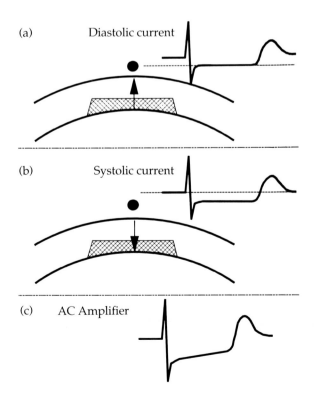

(a)   Diastolic current

(b)   Systolic current

(c)   AC Amplifier

and the magnitude of mechanical tension developed in the ventricular wall during contraction. Increases in any of these parameters raises oxygen demand. Coronary blood flow can be reduced by a chronic arterial obstruction such as that produced by coronary atherosclerosis or thrombosis, or by transient reductions in the diameter of the arterial lumen induced by increases in tone of the muscle in the arterial wall, i.e., vasoconstriction.

4.2.1 Hemodynamic Consequences of Coronary Obstruction

Under normal conditions, blood flow to the ventricular wall rises as oxygen demand increases.[60] For example, during exercise, myocardial blood flow can increase by 600% as heart rate and contractility rise. Myocardial ischemia does not, therefore, develop even though oxygen demand markedly increases. However, in the presence of a coronary artery obstruction, the magnitude of the achievable flow increase is limited. Blood flow at rest may be adequate to meet the needs of the myocardium, but, when oxygen demand during exercise exceeds the ability of flow to increase, myocardial ischemia develops.

Normally, blood flow is evenly distributed across the ventricular wall. Reductions in coronary blood flow or increases in oxygen demand produce a redirection of blood flow away from the inner wall of the ventricles. Epicardial flow is maintained until coronary flow reaches levels near 0. Thus, with both supply-dependent and demand-dependent ischemia, the subendocardium is first jeopardized and subendocardial ischemia develops. Transmural ischemia, with reductions in flow to all layers of the ventricular wall, develops only with more severe reductions in flow.

4.2.2 Electrophysiologic Effects of Myocardial Ischemia

Myocardial ischemia affects cellular electrophysiologic properties in characteristic ways (Figure 4.3).[61] First, the transmembrane resting potential of ischemic cells rises to less negative values and cells are partially depolarized. Resting membrane potentials rise from normal levels of near –90 mV to less negative values of approximately –60 to –65 mV within minutes of coronary occlusion.

Second, action potential duration is shortened. This begins within minutes of coronary blockage and reaches maximal levels within 30 minutes. This abnormality reflects abbreviation of the plateau phase of the action potential waveform as well as an acceleration of the fall in potential during phase 3. Thus, subendocardial ischemia shortens inner wall action potential durations to reverse the normal transmural recovery gradient. The ischemic inner wall now recovers before the normal outer wall (Figure 4.3).

4.2.3 Injury Currents

Partial depolarization and shortened action potential duration generate potential gradients between ischemic and neighboring normal cells.[61] These potential gradients result in flow of injury currents between regions (Figure 4.3).

During phase 4 of the action potential, the intracellular resting potential of ischemic cells is less negative to the more negative normal cells (Figure 4.3). This potential gradient is eliminated when both the ischemic and normal regions are activated and the injury current ceases to flow. Because these currents flow only during electrical diastole, they are termed diastolic injury currents.

The shortening of ischemic action potential duration causes the intracellular potential of ischemic cells to become more negative during phases 2 and 3 than in normal cells. Intracellular positive current then flows from normal to ischemic cells during electrical systole to create systolic injury currents (Figure 4.3). Thus, the direction of the systolic injury current is opposite that of the diastolic injury current.

4.3 *Electrocardiographic Effects of Myocardial Ischemia*

Injury currents can be detected by electrocardiographic leads placed on the body surface. The pattern observed varies, however, depending on the type of ECG amplifier used. A direct, or DC, coupled amplifier commonly operates in standard voltmeters to measure the absolute level of voltage in a circuit. The potential at one electrode is measured in volts relative to a 0 reference or ground potential.

Most clinical ECG systems have a capacitor-coupled stage in the amplifier. Hence, they are known as capacitor coupled, or AC-coupled, amplifier systems. This capacitor prevents conduction of DC current but allows passage of alternating, or AC, current. Because the DC level of the ECG record is eliminated, ECG voltages cannot be measured relative to a segment of the ECG waveform defined as the baseline level. The TP segment (that is, the interval between the end of the P wave and the beginning of the QRS complex) is normally selected as the baseline reference level against which other wave amplitudes are evaluated.

4.3.1 DC-Coupled Amplifiers

Figure 4.4 represents a unipolar ECG electrode over an ischemic zone, connected to a DC-coupled amplifier. Diastolic injury currents flow from ischemic subendocardial cells to normal subepicardial cells, i.e., toward the electrode. They thus produce a positive potential shift in the amplifier output during electrical diastole during the TQ segment (Figure 4.4). The recording returns to baseline levels once depolarization begins and remains at that level until recovery is complete at the end of the T wave.

Systolic currents are directed from normal subepicardial to ischemic subendocardial cells and away from the electrode. They thus generate negative potentials in the ECG waveform during the period of electrical systole, the ST-T interval (Figure 4.4a). The recorded ST segment is depressed. Hence, a DC-coupled ECG recording exhibits TQ segment elevation followed by ST segment depression.

4.3.2 AC-Coupled Amplifier

The rise in the absolute magnitude of TQ segment potentials generated by diastolic injury currents cannot be directly measured in AC-coupled systems because this interval serves as the baseline level. However, because diastolic injury currents cease once ischemic and normal tissue are activated, the ST-T interval occurs at a lower potential level than the TP segment. This appears as relative, or apparent, or secondary ST segment depression in the AC-coupled output.

Systolic injury currents also produce a negative shift in the ST segment. This shift occurs as a direct or primary ST segment depression. Hence, both systolic and diastolic injury currents summate to produce ST segment depression in capacitor-coupled recordings from a unipolar electrode on normal tissue overlying an ischemic zone (Figure 4.4). This ST segment depression results from both primary and secondary ST depression and is the hallmark of subendocardial myocardial ischemia.[61]

4.4 *Recording Electrocardiographic Effects of Myocardial Ischemia*

ST segment analysis can be performed in several clinical settings. First, ST segment abnormalities can be monitored in patients hospitalized in coronary care units, intensive care units, operating rooms, emergency rooms, or similar monitored units. Such patients commonly have unstable angina pectoris, acute myocardial infarction, or recent cardiovascular surgery. Second, ST segment potentials can be computed from long-term (24 to 72 hours) tape recordings of ECG rhythms in ambulatory patients, i.e., long-term electrocardiographic recording or Holter monitoring. Important instrumentation requirements must be met in each clinical setting to ensure accurate recordings.

4.4.1 ECG Lead Systems

Myocardial ischemia generally occurs as a regional event produced by narrowing of a coronary artery that supplies a particular area of the heart. The resulting electrophysiologic abnormalities produce electrocardiographic changes in electrodes topographically related to the injured area. Because lesions can form in vessels supplying any area of the heart, recording electrodes must reside on body surface locations that permit detection of relevant electrocardiographic information from all cardiac regions.

A complete sampling of all cardiac areas would require hundreds of electrodes, a technically impossible situation in most clinical settings. Specific leads can be designed, however, that permit detection of ischemic abnormalities from most large areas of the heart. Leads that sample all three major axes of the cardiac electrical field (anterior-posterior, right-left, and superior-inferior) can detect abnormalities from all cardiac regions.[62] Most commonly, leads approximating lead V_1 or V_2 in the anterior-posterior axis, lead V_5 in the right-left axis, and lead aVF in the superior-inferior axis are best suited for ST segment analysis.[62,63]

Such a lead system may be constructed in coronary care units using electrode locations originally designed for exercise stress tests as depicted in Figure 1.10.[64] The ECG patterns recorded from these leads are very similar to those registered by standard ECG systems. Although many monitoring systems permit surveillance of only one lead at a time, recommendations that two leads be simultaneously monitored have been made.[62] Additional leads may be needed for particular purposes.

For ambulatory monitoring, two leads are commonly recorded (Figure 1.14).[63] One lead, similar to lead V_1, is constructed from electrodes placed on the fourth right intercostal space 1 inch from the sternal margin (positive pole) and on the lateral one-third of the

Figure 4.5–(a) Normal ST-T waves. (b) Development of ST-segment depression that was not associated with pain.

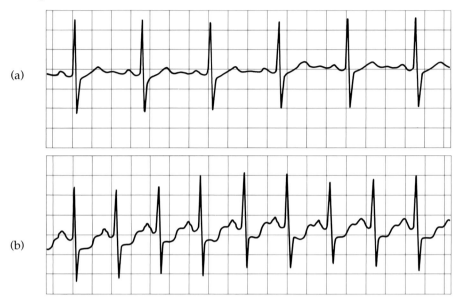

(a)

(b)

Figure 4.6–Ranges of prevalences of transient ST-segment shifts for various clinical forms of coronary artery disease, based upon literature from 1965 through 1989.

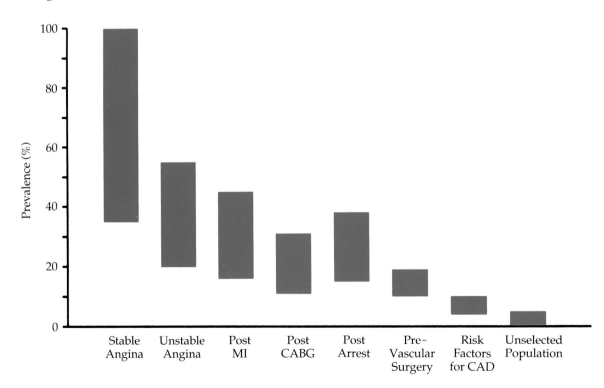

left infraclavicular fossa (negative pole) and 1 inch below the inferior angle of the right scapula on the posterior torso (negative electrode).

4.4.2 Amplifier and Monitor Systems

Electronic characteristics of the amplifier and associated hardware are critically important for the recording of ST segment abnormalities. The ST segment has a frequency content considerably lower than that of the QRS complex. Hence, particular attention must be given to all components that can attenuate low frequency interference. These components include patient-related elements, electrode systems, and amplifiers.

The major patient-related elements are respiration and body motion. Low-frequency chest wall movements cause baseline wander that can either mimic or obscure true transient ST segment shifts. Inadequate skin preparation before attaching electrodes and insecure electrode placement can also increase electrode interface noise to cause excessive baseline drift. Optimal recordings require applying electrodes away from muscular areas and bony prominences to reduce motion artifacts. Cleaning the skin with alcohol and mild abrasives removes oils and dead layers of cells that increase impedance. Final measured impedance should measure less than 5000 ohms, and preferably less than 3500 ohms.[62,63]

Amplifier characteristics are critical, especially frequency response and phase response. The common low-frequency limit of monitoring amplifiers of 0.5 Hz can significantly distort the ST segment and may artifactually produce ST segment shifts.[65,66] Using the same low-frequency cutoff of 0.05 Hz recommended for diagnostic electrocardiographs is best.[67] Strict adherence to this requirement can, however, cause so much baseline wander it makes the monitor useless. A system with an amplitude response that is flat to a few tenths of 1.0 Hz may be adequate if linearity between phase shift and frequency response is maintained. Specific recommendations of a task force of the American Heart Association, for example, include an amplitude response that is flat to within 0.5 decibel (dB) to 1.0 Hz and a −3 dB cutoff of less than 0.33 Hz if the system has a phase response at least as good as a linear 0.05 Hz single-pole amplifier system.[62] Frequency modulated (FM) tape recorder systems with frequency responses flat to essentially 0.0 Hz are not required.

4.4.3 Analysis Systems

Virtually all ST segment analysis systems rely on computerized processing of the ECG signal. Automated analysis systems must accurately detect all significant ST segment shifts (i.e., have high sensitivity) without including artifact (i.e., have high specificity). Several specific conditions should be met by these systems. The automated system must select an appropriate baseline period (usually during the TP segment or PR segment) and identify the end of the QRS complex (the J point) to accurately quantify the potential at a particular instant during the ST segment. Most systems allow the user to specify the exact baseline and analysis time points. The ST segment shifts should likewise be used only on normally conducted complexes and not on ectopic beats.

Finally, it cannot be overemphasized that the clinical effectiveness of the monitoring system depends on the expertise of the user regardless of the sophistication of the hardware and software. Adequate and recurrent training of technical, as well as professional, staff remains absolutely essential for successful operation in a clinical environment.

4.5 Electrocardiographic Features of Transient Ischemia

Ischemic ST segments, characteristically depressed, are horizontal or flat in shape (Figure 4.5). The ST depression can occur with or without T wave inversion. The T waves can be inverted in the absence of ST segment depression. Diagnostic criteria for an ischemic episode require 0.1 mV of flat or downsloping ST segment depression 80 msec after the J point that lasts 60 to 90 seconds or longer. Such flat depression is rare in normal subjects. Less commonly, ST segment elevation occurs rather than depression, and is largely limited to patients with unstable angina pectoris or acute myocardial infarction.

Most episodes last less than 5 minutes, although some can last several hours. The number of episodes per day varies widely. In patients with stable angina pectoris, for example, ischemic episodes number up to 25 per day with a total duration of 1 to over 400 minutes per 24-hour period.[68] A marked increase in frequency occurs during the first two to four waking hours of the day.[69]

4.6 Clinical Significance of Transient ST Segment Depression

Ischemic ST depression can be detected in most patients with coronary artery disease and in a very small minority of healthy subjects.[70] It is particularly common in patients with stable and unstable angina and in those experiencing the onset of acute myocardial infarction (Figure 4.6).

The presence of ST segment shifts on ambulatory ECG has a high specificity (over 90%) but only a moderate sensitivity (37% to 54%) for identifying patients with underlying coronary artery disease.[68,70] Many episodes of transient ischemia occur during physical and mental activity.[71] The incidence is greater during more intense activities. For example, performing various forms of mental arithmetic is particularly provocative. However, many episodes develop at rest or with only mild exertion. Transient ischemia begins by either increases in oxygen demand produced by rises in heart rate or blood pressure or by decreases in myocardial blood flow produced by vasoconstriction.[72]

Most episodes are not associated with symptoms, and thus they represent silent myocardial ischemia.[73] In patients with stable angina pectoris, over 85% of episodes are painless and approximately 45% of patients have only painless ischemia. Hypotheses have been proposed explaining why most episodes do not produce pain. This mechanism may be particularly relevant in diabetics with peripheral neuropathy. A greater percentage of these patients have only silent episodes than do other patient populations. The degree of ischemia during painless episodes can be less than during painful attacks. Painful episodes last longer, are associated with greater ST segment depression, and, in some studies, cause greater left ventricular dysfunction than painless ones.

As many as one third of patients with transient ST segment depression develop ventricular arrhythmias during the ischemic episodes.[74] Patients with arrhythmias have more frequent ischemic episodes, longer episodes with ectopy, and greater ST depression than other episodes.

Myocardial ischemia—whether symptomatic or asymptomatic—is an important prognostic factor in patients with stable angina pectoris. The incidence of death, infarction, unstable angina, or need for surgical revascularization is much greater in patients with ECG evidence of transient ischemia.[75]

In patients with unstable angina, the total duration of ischemic ST depression directly correlates with extent of coronary artery disease and with development of acute infarction or death. Patients with over 60 minutes of ischemia per day have a particularly poor outcome; over 90% develop acute infarction or require revascularization.[76]

Similarly, the presence of transient ischemic episodes during the early or late postinfarction period is a poor prognostic sign.[77,78] Recurrent infarction occurs more commonly in those with ischemia during hospitalization. Patients with ischemic ST segment shifts after infarction have a much higher prevalence of death, reinfarction, or unstable angina than those without ischemia. Thus, transient ischemia indicates a poor prognosis in all forms of symptomatic coronary artery disease.

Finally, transient ischemic ECG changes during the preoperative and early postoperative period after noncardiac surgery is a poor prognostic sign.[79] These changes are most frequent after vascular surgery and on the third postoperative day. Severe postoperative ischemic complications, including unstable angina, infarction, and death, occur almost only in patients with ischemic episodes; patients with postoperative ischemia have over a nine-fold greater risk of such events than do those without transient ischemia.

5.0 PEDIATRIC ELECTROCARDIOGRAPHY

Pediatric arrhythmias have some similarities in the electrocardiographic appearance and subsequent interpretation to adult electrocardiographic characteristics. However, differences in the underlying substrate, clinical presentation, electrocardiographic appearance, and subsequent therapy of many pediatric arrhythmias remain important.

This section describes some of the electrocardiographic differences between children and adults that have direct bearing on age-appropriate electrocardiogram (ECG) interpretation.

5.1 *Heart Rate*

One of the most elementary diagnoses made from the surface ECG is that of heart rate. This simple interpretation can become a quagmire for the observer unaccustomed to the developmental spectrum of normal heart rates seen in infants and children. The range of "normal" heart rates varies as a function of age, presumably due to both postnatal adaptations to circulatory changes and the plasticity of cardiovascular control by the autonomic nervous system (Table 5.1).

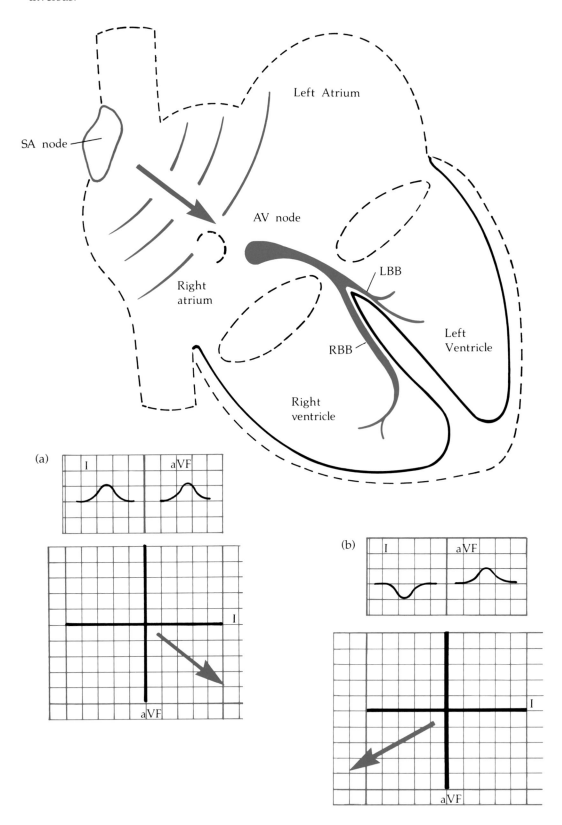

Figure 5.1–(a) Abnormal situs solitus. (b) Atrial situs inversus.

SA node

Left Atrium

AV node

Right atrium

LBB

RBB

Left Ventricle

Right ventricle

(a)

I   aVF

I

aVF

(b)

I   aVF

I

aVF

Table 5.1— Normal heart rates in children.

Age	Mean Heart Rate (in bpm)	Range
First day	123	93-154
First week	126	91-166
2-4 weeks	148	107-182
1-2 months	149	121-179
3-5 months	141	106-186
6-11 months	134	109-169
1-2 years	119	89-151
3-4 years	108	73-137
5-7 years	100	65-133
8-11 years	91	62-130
12-15 years	85	60-119

The normal mean heart rate increases from 120 bpm at birth to 150 bpm by the end of the second month of life. However, infants can manifest sinus tachycardia to 200 to 210 bpm during crying, fever, or serious illnesses. Heart rate gradually declines back to a mean of 120 bpm by 1 to 2 years of age and to 85 bpm in the toddler and early adolescent. Incorrect diagnoses of sinus or supraventricular tachycardias frequently occur when adult standards are applied to infants and children.

5.2 *Intervals and Leads*

Just as pediatric heart rates differ from those of adults, pediatric electrocardiographic intervals differ as well. This fact partially results from a smaller cardiac mass (and therefore shorter time for transmission of electrical impulses) but also from differences in autonomic control of heart rate and blood pressure. The length of the PR interval varies with the patient's age. The mean values in infants would generally be short by adult criteria. Likewise, QRS durations considered normal in the adult, such as 90 to 100 milliseconds, can represent pathologic ventricular conduction defects or ventricular arrhythmias in infants and young children.

In adult patients, the ECG typically consists of 12 leads (I, II, III, aVR, aVL, aVF, V_1-V_6). Pediatric patients require two additional right chest leads, V_3R and V_4R, and a more lateral left chest lead, V_7, resulting in a 15-lead tracing. The additional leads permit adequate investigation of the right ventricle, which can be more dominant in younger children, and the left ventricle and septum, especially in patients with suspected congenital cardiac defects.

5.3 *Cardiac Malposition*

The presence of the cardiac mass in an abnormal position in the chest is generally thought to be a *secondary* manifestation of an extracardiac process. Examples include

Figure 5.2–Ventricular inversion.

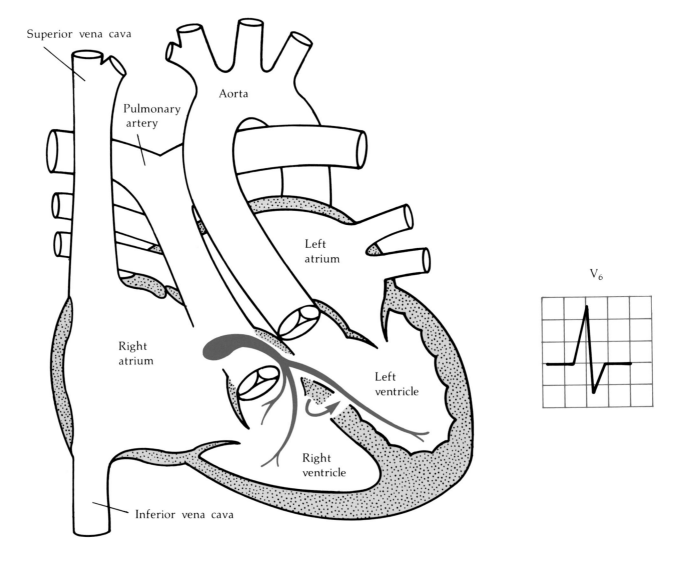

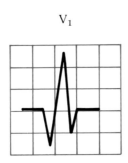

pneumothorax, pneumonectomy, pectus excavatum, kyphoscoliosis, and lung hypoplasia. Many forms of congenital cardiac defects also present with concomitant *primary* cardiac malpositions. These malpositions may involve the atria or ventricles, alone or in combination.

In most cases of abdominal situs solitus (the liver and inferior vena cava on the right side, the spleen and abdominal aorta on the left), the atria are concordant and the normal P wave vector reflects the spread of activation from the high right atrium to the left and downward (Figure 5.1a). However, when atrial situs inversus occurs, the resulting P wave is negative in lead I and positive in lead aVF (Figure 5.1b).

Several types of congenital cardiac defects may also present with abnormalities of ventricular position. With normal ventricular position, the bulk of the ventricular mass consists of left ventricular myocardium and is located to the left and inferior. Again, age-dependent changes occur in ventricular mass, especially in the neonatal period, that result in differing R and S wave amplitudes in the precordial chest leads. The major cause is the change from a relative hypertrophy of the newborn right ventricle in the first weeks of life (reflecting in utero pressure volume relationships) to a dominant left ventricular mass.

The electrocardiographic definition of "dextrocardia" requires the presence of greater voltage (R plus S) in the right chest leads V_3R or V_4R than the transitional chest leads V_3 or V_4. This results from the greater cardiac mass being located in the right side of the chest. A recording of full right chest leads, V_3R through V_7R, should be made in this situation.

Other manifestations of ventricular malpositions include "reversed" septal depolarization with initial septal Q waves in the right chest leads and absent Q waves on the left. The reversal can result from ventricular inversion, in which the morphologic left ventricle lies on the right side receiving blood from the right atrium and pumping to the pulmonary artery. The right ventricle resides on the left, receiving blood from the left atrium and emptying into the aorta (Figure 5.2). The condition is also called l-transposition of the great arteries or "corrected" transposition. The conduction system "travels" with the ventricles, so septal depolarization proceeds from left ventricle to right ventricle, and from right to left on the surface ECG. The septal Q wave therefore is noted in the right precordial leads.

5.4   *Effects of Congenital Heart Defects*

The entire spectrum of congenital malformations of the heart is too broad to review in this section. The reader should consult several excellent textbooks on the subject.[80-82] However, notable examples of structural congenital heart defects result in specific electrocardiographic abnormalities that warrant discussion.

Structural congenital heart defects can occur in an abundance or paucity of cardiac mass. In the newborn infant, several specific ECG findings can point toward specific diagnoses. For example, many defects can result in a relative underdevelopment of the left ventricle in utero (hypoplastic left heart syndrome)(Figure 5.3a). The ECG then shows a paucity of left-sided ventricular forces. Leftward deviation of the frontal plane QRS axis (0 to –90°) in a newborn with Down's syndrome highly suggests the presence of an atrioventricular septal defect (AV canal defect). Left axis deviation in an infant with cyanosis can indicate the presence of tricuspid atresia (Figure 5.3b). In this condition, left axis deviation in AV canal defect can develop from elongation of fibers of the left anterior fascicle or shortening of the left posterior fascicle. Left axis in tricuspid atresia may be due to hypertrophy of the basal portion of the left ventricle.

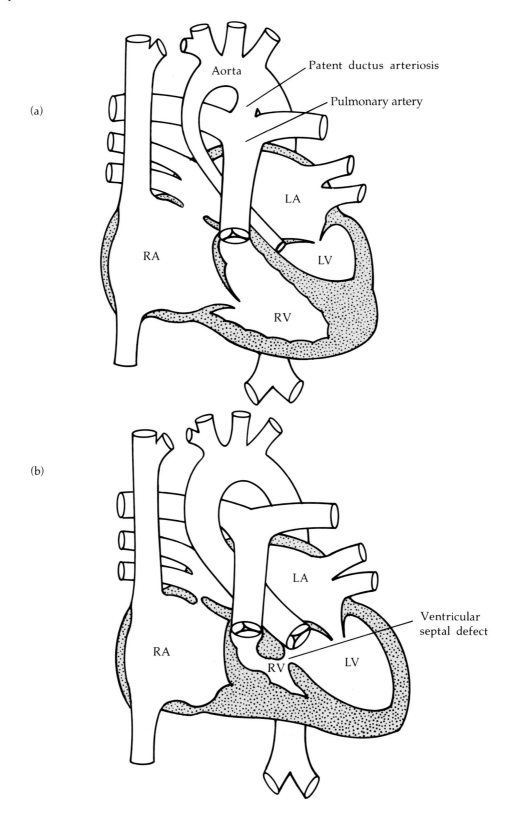

Figure 5.3–(a) Hypoplastic left heart syndrome
(b) Tricuspid atresia.

(a)

Aorta

Patent ductus arteriosis

Pulmonary artery

LA

RA

LV

RV

(b)

LA

RA

Ventricular
septal defect

RV

LV

5.5   *Pediatric Arrhythmias*

5.5.1   Fetal Arrhythmias

The diagnosis and management of fetal cardiac arrhythmias is a relatively new area in pediatric cardiology. Currently, diagnosis of fetal arrhythmias is done using fetal Doppler echocardiography, rather than true fetal electrocardiographic interpretation.[83] The ability to diagnose fetal arrhythmias depends on two essential points: determination of cardiac rate and analysis of rhythm. Doppler echocardiography can yield fetal ventricular inflow and outflow velocity patterns which imply atrial and ventricular contraction, respectively. Interval analysis of these flow patterns is then used to deduce the underlying atrial and ventricular relationships during tachycardia and arrive at an assumed "electrocardiographic" diagnosis. Obtaining simultaneous flow patterns is often difficult and diagnosis becomes one of making the "best guess".

Fetal bradycardia generally is defined as a rate below 100 bpm and tachycardia as a rate consistently above 220 bpm. Other echocardiographic findings helpful in determining the severity of fetal arrhythmias include pericardial effusion, chamber dilation, hypertrophy, prolonged periods of bradycardia, and other evidence of hydrops that reflect in-utero congestive heart failure (for example, ascites, scalp edema, and decreased fetal movement).

Obviously, one would rather obtain a direct fetal cardiac electrical signal to diagnose fetal arrhythmias. The problems in this area are many, predominantly due to the small amplitude of fetal cardiac electrical potentials and fetal position and movement.[84,85] The maternal cardiac signal can be eliminated by means of blanking or subtraction. Filtering of the overall signal to eliminate unwanted noise can distort the lower amplitude and low frequency components of the fetal signal as well, so the end result is suboptimal. Further research is required to make fetal electrocardiography a practical and applicable tool for the pediatric cardiologist.

Using fetal Doppler echocardiography, one can reliably diagnose premature atrial and ventricular contractions, atrial flutter/atrial tachycardia, complete atrioventricular block, supraventricular tachycardia with a 1:1 atrial ventricular relationship, and junctional/ventricular tachycardia. Although interval measurements can discriminate between accessory pathway tachycardias and atrioventricular node reentry tachycardia, a precise determination of the mechanism of the many types of supraventricular tachycardias is not possible using Doppler alone.

5.5.2   Chaotic Atrial Tachycardia

Chaotic atrial tachycardia is an infantile arrhythmia that, when manifested, atrial rates range from 200 to 500 bpm (Figure 5.4). Multiple P wave morphologies and the rhythm can appear as atrial ectopic tachycardia, rapid atrial flutter, and atrial fibrillation all in the same patient. High-grade atrioventricular block is a frequent finding, but ventricular rates can still be very fast. The arrhythmia appears to be a transient phenomenon, disappearing by 18 months of age in the majority of patients. Though difficult to treat, class IC antiarrhythmic agents appear to be most efficacious.[86,87] The cause and mechanism of the arrhythmia are unknown, but it may be secondary to an "atrial myocarditis" or due to changes in the ability of atrial muscle to initiate and maintain rapid tachyarrhythmias at

Figure 5.4–Chaotic atrial tachycardia in a 4-month old.

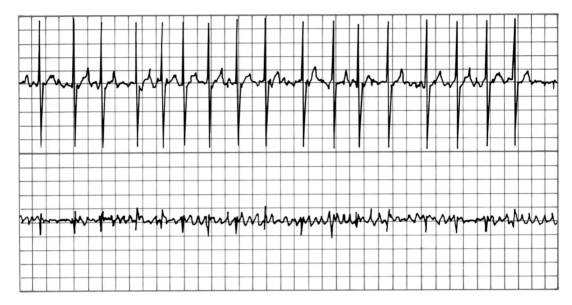

Figure 5.5–Premature atrial contractions (PACs) in a
newborn infant.

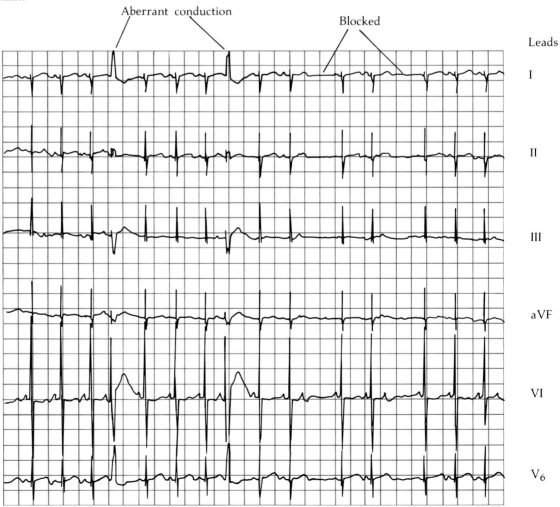

Figure 5.6–Congenital complete atrioventricular block with a narrow QRS (junctional rhythm).

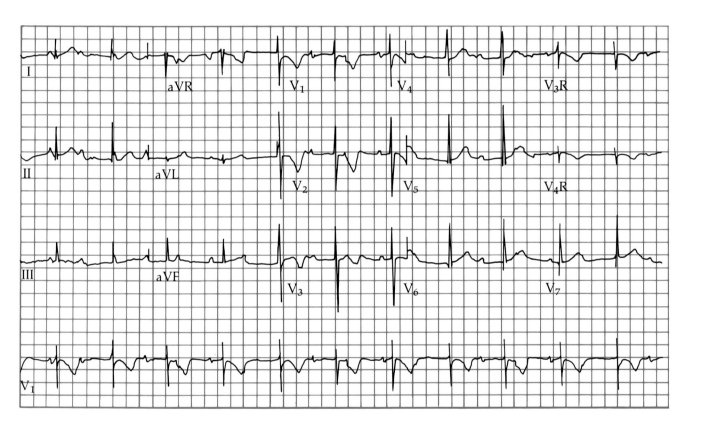

Figure 5.7–(a) Sinus bradycardia with a very long QT interval and bizarre T waves. (b) T wave alternans (nearly diagnostic of long QT syndrome) in the same patient.

(a)

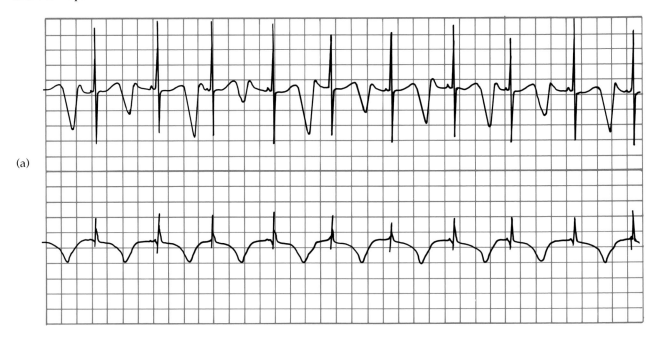

(b)

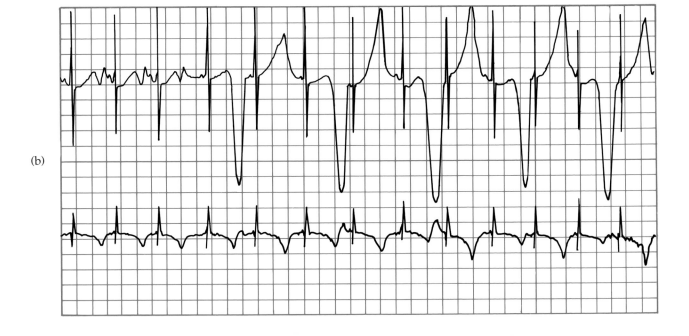

various stages of development. The ECG manifestations of chaotic atrial tachycardia blur the distinctions between classic notions of automatic, triggered, macrore-entrant and microre-entrant arrhythmias.

5.5.3   Bradycardia in the Newborn

The diagnosis of sinus bradycardia is age dependent. The newborn with a heart rate of 70 or 80 bpm may have sinus bradycardia, whereas this is a perfectly acceptable heart rate for an adult. As a rough guide, potentially significant bradycardia consists of less than 70 bpm for an infant, less than 50 bpm for a child, and less than 40 bpm for an adolescent. The P waves should have the standard frontal plane axis of 0 to 90° to infer a sinus mechanism (assuming a normal heart).

Bradycardia in the newborn nursery is a frequent cause of concern. The most common cause is blocked premature atrial contractions (PACs). A careful inspection for P waves "hidden" in the T waves often is necessary and requires a full 15-lead ECG (Figure 5.5). Bedside monitor strips are inadequate for appropriate diagnosis. The overwhelming majority of blocked PACs resolve without therapy or symptoms.

Congenital complete AV block (CCAVB) consists of independent atrial and ventricular rhythms (Figure 5.6). Up to 25% of patients with this rhythm also have prolongation of the corrected QT interval and can have a higher risk of sudden death.[88] In approximately one third of cases of CCAVB, an underlying congenital cardiac malformation exists, such as l-transposition of the great arteries, "single ventricle", atrioventricular septal defects, tricuspid atresia and coarctation. In the infant with a normal heart, a relationship can occur between CCAVB and overt maternal collagen vascular disease (lupus erythematosus) or positive serum assays for maternal antibodies (anti-Rho).[89] Histochemical evidence for the presence of these antibodies in AV node tissue and disruption of the AV node-bundle of His region have been found.

As stated earlier, CCAVB can be diagnosed in the fetus. Ventricular rates with CCAVB vary from one patient to the next and in individuals, depending on autonomic tone. Escape rates can be junctional or ventricular. Generally, ventricular rates under 50 bpm in an infant necessitate placement of an epicardial pacing system. Some stressed infants require pacing despite more rapid ventricular rates (55 to 60 bpm). Pacing for the fetus with CCAVB may be necessary because of hydrops and either prematurity or too great a risk of delivery. Investigations are underway to develop a maternal transabdominal fetal epicardial pacing system.

Careful measurement of the corrected QT interval (QTc = QT/RR) must be made in the infant with sinus bradycardia, since bradycardia is a frequent finding in newborns with long QT syndrome (Figure 5.7). Additionally, a 2:1 AV block may be present. These patients are at risk for ventricular tachycardia, ventricular fibrillation, and torsade de pointes (Figure 5.8).

Figure 5.8–Torsade de pointes ventricular tachycardia.

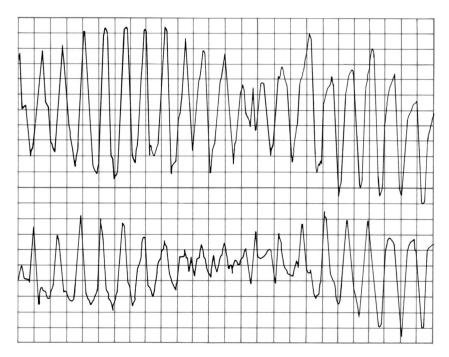

Figure 5.9–Congenital junctional ectopic tachycardia (JET).

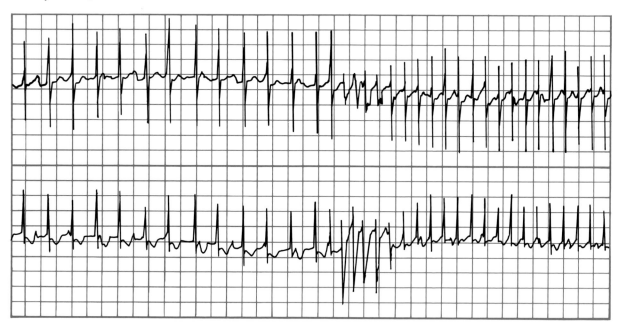

5.5.4 Developmental Aspects of Wolff-Parkinson-White Syndrome and Supraventricular Tachycardia

Supraventricular tachycardia (SVT) associated with an accessory connection is the most common mechanism of SVT in childhood. Many reports suggest that Wolff-Parkinson-White syndrome (WPW) and SVT disappear in the first year of life. Others report that SVT recurs sometime later.

The clinical course of 140 patients with SVT and WPW was reviewed at Texas Children's Hospital.[90] Among patients whose SVT appeared at 0 to 2 months of age, it disappeared in 93% by 8 months of age. In nearly one third of these 93%, it reappeared at an average age of 8 years. If SVT occurred in a patient over the age of 5 years, it persisted in more than 75%. The location of the accessory connection did not affect the recurrence rate. Additionally, the age at recurrence was not affected by concomitant antiarrhythmic drug therapy.

These findings lend credence to the notion that autonomic or hormonal changes in the mechanisms of cardiovascular control affect the time course of SVT in young patients. The mean age of SVT recurrence is similar to that at which the symptom complex of mitral valve prolapse first appears, vasodepressor syncope begins to emerge, and T waves invert in the right precordial leads.

5.5.5 Junctional Ectopic Tachycardia

Junctional ectopic tachycardia (JET) can be either congenital or acquired following surgery for congenital heart defects. Mortality rates for congenital JET are very high (approximately 33%) despite aggressive therapy.[91] The surface ECG usually is characteristic: rapid, narrow QRS complexes at 150 to 400 bpm with atrioventricular dissociation. However, JET can also manifest "exit block" with sudden 1:1 conduction and rates greater than 300 bpm (Figure 5.9). If occasional sinus beats occur, the surface QRS morphology should be similar to that seen during tachycardia, otherwise a diagnosis of ventricular tachycardia is made.

The underlying mechanism of JET remains unclear, but appears to involve abnormal automaticity. The therapy of congenital JET is controversial. High dose amiodarone, class IC antiarrhythmic drugs, and pacing have been used with varying success.

5.5.6 Permanent Junctional Reciprocating Tachycardia

Permanent junctional reciprocating tachycardia (PJRT) is an incessant SVT found in young children.[92-94] As its name implies, it does not disappear with age. The ECG during PJRT shows a long R-P tachyarrhythmia with characteristic deep and inverted P waves in leads II, III, aVF, and the left precordial leads V_4-V_6 (Figure 5.10). The rate of PJRT varies through the day and with activity, but is generally in the range of 150 to 180 bpm. The PJRT results in a secondary cardiomyopathy.

Although the ECG manifestation of PJRT is quite remarkable, four other tachyarrhythmias can have a similar appearance: a low atrial ectopic tachycardia, "atypical" (fast-

Figure 5.10–Permanent junctional reciprocating tachycardia (PJRT).

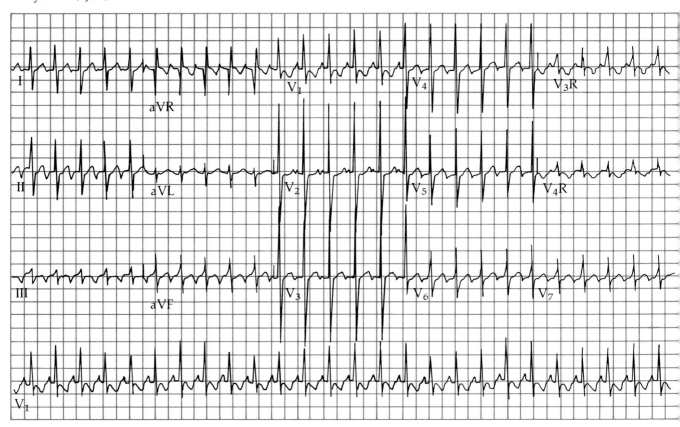

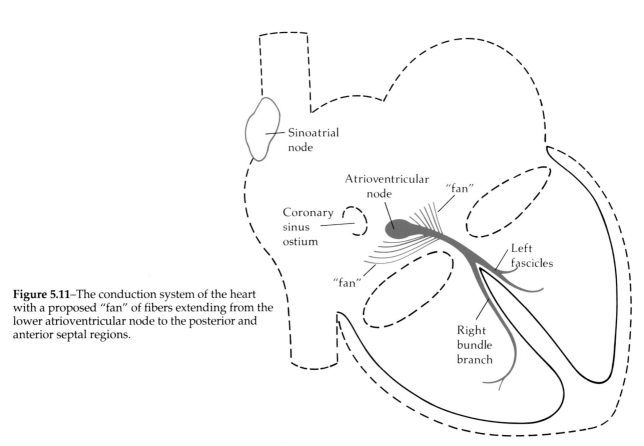

Figure 5.11–The conduction system of the heart with a proposed "fan" of fibers extending from the lower atrioventricular node to the posterior and anterior septal regions.

slow) atrioventricular node re-entry tachycardia, atrial flutter with 2:1 AV conduction, and SVT using a slowly conducting retrograde pathway in the right anterior region of the heart.

Electrophysiologic studies and operative mapping techniques have localized the atrial insertion point of the retrograde fiber to the mouth of the coronary sinus. Pathology examinations have revealed a serpiginous fiber in this region in one patient.[93] The actual mechanism of tachycardia may involve a spectrum of SVTs from "atypical" AV node re-entry to PJRT due to a "fan" of fibers with variable retrograde conduction spanning the posterior septal-AV node area (Figure 5.11). The tachycardia responds to Class IC antiarrhythmic drugs, operative therapy (cryoablation of the retrograde limb) or, more recently, transcatheter radio frequency ablation.[86,95,96]

5.5.7 Ventricular Tachycardia

Infant VT is a rare condition and is most often associated with ventricular hamartomas.[97] The VT in infants can present, disturbingly, as a very rapid rhythm with a narrow QRS of 80 to 100 milliseconds (Figure 5.12). The diagnosis depends on demonstration of a different QRS complex during sinus beats on the 15-lead ECG. The most common picture is one of a right bundle branch block pattern with left-axis deviation associated with a tumor (hamartoma or Purkinje cell tumor) in the posterior left ventricle.[18]

The child with a congenital heart defect has a very good chance of not only surviving initial cardiac repair of the defect, but of having an excellent hemodynamic result. As these children grow, however, many develop late postoperative arrhythmias and an appreciable incidence of late sudden death results following repair of particular lesions.[98-101] Speculation has pointed toward the development of myocardial scars (both atrial and ventricular) to account for the substrate of tachycardia. Lesions prone to late postoperative arrhythmia include tetralogy of Fallot, double outlet right ventricle, ventricular septal defect, aortic valve stenosis, transposition of the great arteries, and Ebstein's malformation of the tricuspid valve.

The mechanisms underlying postoperative arrhythmias are unknown. However, triggered ectopy may initiate the sustained re-entrant arrhythmias. The underlying scar can provide the necessary myocardial inhomogeneity with autonomic changes around the time of adolescence contributing as well.

5.5.8 Permanent Pacing Systems in Children

A complete discussion of pediatric issues in cardiac pacing is beyond the scope of this section. References are provided for the interested reader.[102-104] However, several important points can be made.

The first issue is that of life-long pacing. In adults, the placing of a permanent pacing system considers an additional 20 years of life expectancy. In children, the requirements for adequate cardiac pacing can span more than 50 to 60 years. Therefore, generator battery life (and how to prolong it as much as possible), the effects of growth on lead position, the ability to remove and replace leads after several years use, reuse of pacemaker pockets and venous access, size of both generators and leads in smaller patients, and the changing heart rate requirements during normal growth and development must be considered. The

Figure 5.12–Ventricular tachycardia in an infant. There is AV dissociation and a QRS duration of 70 to 90 milliseconds.

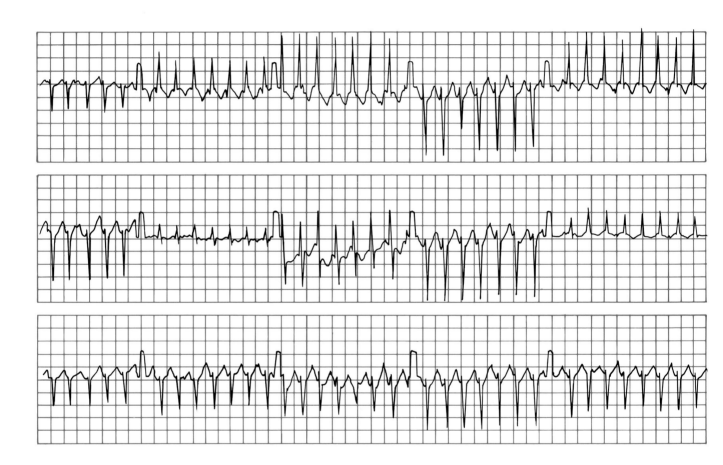

indications for implanting permanent pacing systems therefore cannot be simple extensions of those formulated for adult patients.

5.6 *Pediatric Electrophysiology Studies*

Biplane fluoroscopy is essential to performing pediatric electrophysiologic (EP) studies safely. The infant or child's heart is dramatically smaller than that of an adult and very slight manipulation of an intracardiac catheter can result in large catheter position changes and potential cardiac perforation. Biplane fluoroscopy allows instantaneous localization of the catheter tip and safe movement within the heart and vessels.

Sedation is an additional consideration. Even adolescents typically cannot remain still for adequate intracardiac electrogram recording and smaller children often require heavy sedation. The effect of sedative agents on the desired EP measurements must be taken into account, since conduction and recovery times can be altered significantly. The continuous measurement of the blood pressure is an important part of pediatric EP studies. Small children can develop significant hypotension during induction of tachyarrhythmias.

Manipulation of electrode catheters within the heart requires training in pediatric electrophysiology. Special catheters for pediatric EP studies generally are 5 or 6 French diameter with electrodes spaced 2 or 5 mm apart. Size 4 French catheters often are used in infants.

Since mapping of left-heart structures occasionally becomes imperative for investigation of atrial ectopic tachycardias and VTs (beyond a simple coronary sinus approach), use of the transseptal technique is helpful, especially in children. Mapping of these areas in adults generally occurs by a retrograde arterial approach. This approach is neither safe nor practical in children, due to the smaller caliber of the femoral artery and the greatly increased potential for postcatheterization arterial complications. The transseptal approach allows access to the left atrium and left ventricle without damage to the femoral artery. The use of a "steerable" EP catheter generally permits extensive left-heart mapping from this approach.

The indications for pediatric EP study vary from institution to institution.[105] Those currently used at Texas Children's Hospital are shown in Table 5.2. With the development of radio frequency techniques for the elimination of tachyarrhythmias, these indications are changing rapidly.

Table 5.2—Indications for pediatric electrophysiology study.

1. Map accessory connection(s) in patient with SVT to:
   a. Estimate risk to patient during atrial fibrillation,
   b. Prepare for surgical intervention,
   c. Perform radiofrequency ablation.
2. Determine mechanism of unknown type of SVT.
3. Map atrial ectopic focus for surgery or ablation.
4. Map VT focus for surgery or ablation.
5. Determine mechanism of wide QRS tachycardia.
6. Determine drug efficacy for tachyarrhythmias.
7. Assess conduction properties, blood pressure response to pacing prior to pacemaker implantation.
8. Determine presence of occult arrhythmia in patient with syncope.
9. Ablation of junctional ectopic tachycardia.
10. Map site of atrioventricular block (rarely necessary).
11. Investigational study of postoperative patients.
12. Ablation of atrial flutter (future).
13. Overdrive pacing of tachyarrhythmia.

6.0 HEART RATE VARIABILITY

Heart rate variability (HRV) has received recent attention as a noninvasive indicator of the relative balance of parasympathetic and sympathetic influences on the heart. Areas of clinical interest in which the central autonomic nervous system (CANS) may play a role can sometimes benefit from quantitative HRV assessment. HRV has been used to measure maturation in fetuses and neonates, and has contributed to an understanding of sudden infant death syndrome (SIDS). Autonomic neuropathy, brainstem status, brain death, and coma also have been evaluated with HRV. The staging of diabetic neuropathy using HRV methods is particularly well developed. In addition to elucidating cardiorespiratory interactions, simple HRV measures have proven sensitive as specific empirical risk indices in hypertension, acute myocardial infarction (AMI), congestive heart failure (CHF), and sudden cardiac death (SCD). The psychobiological mechanisms underlying the effects of psychological stress, trait coping predispositions, cognitive demands, and affective experience can also be explored using this noninvasive technique.

Part of the appeal of HRV is the ease of collection of heart rate (HR) information in laboratory, clinical, and naturalistic situations. The recent developments in Holter technology has made it practical and economical to monitor electrocardiogram (ECG) parameters such as the R-to-R interval (the inverse of the instantaneous HR) over periods of days in ambulatory subjects with a noninvasive and relatively comfortable preparation. High quality HR data results from a wide variety of modern clinical data collection systems, particularly those found in well-developed intensive or coronary care facilities.

The term "arrhythmia" often carries negative connotations, and indeed many serious disturbances of heart rhythm and waveform morphology are so labeled. However, the novice clinician soon learns that some arrhythmias are normal in healthy subjects. In fact, a moderate amount of respiratory sinus arrhythmia (RSA) is viewed as evidence of good cardiovascular health. An RSA is a particular patterned sequence of changes in heart interbeat interval that is coupled in a complex way to respiratory behavior. The coupling is mediated by central autonomic neural mechanisms of theoretical and clinical interest.

Physiology textbooks, emphasizing principles of homeostasis, often imply that a well-regulated system is always one with minimal variation, and that fluctuations in HR, particularly when metabolic demand appears constant, are undesirable. However, regulating HR at a precise constant value may be less beneficial than maintaining tight control of blood pressure. Also, maintaining the capacity for responsive control of blood pressure to body areas critical for life under the most adverse metabolic, vasostatic, and psychologic conditions appears more adaptive. HR is an intervening variable in homeostatic control loops in the body, its general regulation an incidental consequence of more pervasive optimization criteria.

At the most basic level, HRV is the beat-by-beat change in the length of each heart interbeat interval. Statistical characterization of HRV ranges from measures of distributional spread like the familiar standard deviation to the cutting edge of methods research in nonstationary multivariate time-series analysis. Under ideal conditions, time series and power spectral analyses of the R-to-R interval sequence allow the fractionation of the effects of sympathetic and parasympathetic influences on the heart rhythm. These analyses effectively identify and quantify RSA, a mode of variability considered almost purely parasympathetic in origin. The HR signal is very sensitive to perturbation from many biological and psychological sources. Statistical properties of the dynamic state of the HR may provide noninvasive indices of central autonomic function, a theoretically important, but generally difficult, dimension in many comprehensive health science models.

This section reviews some of the better known measures for heart rhythm analysis and discusses the practical issues associated with their implementation. Simple systems models of the physiology of the innervation of the heart are introduced and the basic concepts of instantaneous heart period (HP) and HR are defined. Issues related to the choice of HR or HP as the fundamental unit of analysis are explored, with the distinctions between time-weighted versus beat-weighted statistical summaries addressed. A variety of HRV measures relevant to 24-hour ambulatory Holter ECG monitoring include variance-based measures, magnitude of change measures, and spectral analysis approaches. Four types of spectral analysis exist, depending on the decision to analyze the HP data sequences in real time or in beat time and to use traditional nonparametric Fourier spectral estimates or parametric autoregressive model-based spectral estimates.

The application of nonlinear dynamic systems analysis techniques to empirical HRV data, including chaos theory approaches, is briefly discussed. The most serious problem in HRV analysis may relate to the identification, labeling, and appropriate treatment of nonsinus beats. A number of other issues regarding the validity and comparability of HRV measures in realistic clinical settings are also described.

Figure 6.1–Simplified model used in the interpretation of heart rate variability statistics

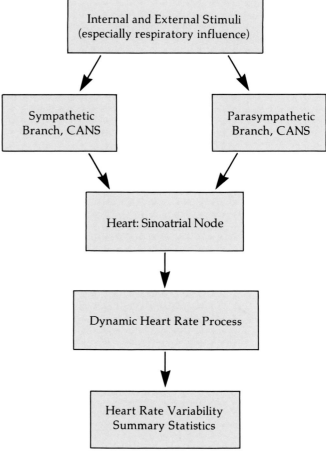

Figure 6.2–Comparison of the 24-hour dynamic heart period sequence in a normal subject and a post-transplant heart patient.

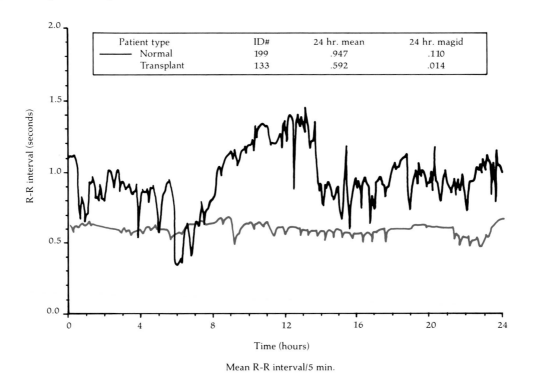

Patient type	ID#	24 hr. mean	24 hr. magid
Normal	199	.947	.110
Transplant	133	.592	.014

Mean R-R interval/5 min.

6.1 Physiologic Models for Heart Rate Variability Analysis

Interpretation of HRV studies is based on a simple model of the initiation of the heart beat. It assumes that dynamic variations in the "normal" beats represent the influence of exogenous and endogenous stimuli on the sinoatrial node, as mediated by the CANS. The statistics of normal heart rhythm can then serve as an indirect indicator of modulation of the inputs to the CANS, the gross function of the CANS itself, or a combination of the two. The model is used to interpret the spectral analysis-based HRV measures because it describes the independent influence on the sinoatrial node of the anatomically distinct sympathetic and parasympathetic branches of the CANS (Figure 6.1). The relative balance of these autonomic mediators is of theoretical interest in clinical cardiology.

Since the impinging neural sources of variation and CANS transfer characteristics cannot be independently isolated with current noninvasive techniques, careful experimental controls or averaging heuristics must be employed to make separate inferences about these domains from the observable heart rhythm data. However, significant perturbation of the stimuli field or neural function can be easily interpreted. For example, phasic psychological stressors and diabetic neuropathy are associated with consistent heart rhythm modifications. Figure 6.2 illustrates the radical extremes of CANS control of the heart, contrasting the large-scale HR variation of the normal subject with the rigidity of the heart rhythm of the post-heart transplant patient.

The model glosses over many details, including the specialized structure of the CANS, interactions with the broader autonomic nervous system, and its influence on the periphery, basic cardiac mechanics of preload and afterload, blood pressure, temperature, respiration, acid-base balance, state of oxygenation, ventilation, physical activity, psychosocial context, and normally mediated facilitating mechanisms. The model implies that a large portion of the endogenous variations result from feedback control mechanisms (e.g., blood pressure control) in which the CANS and/or the heart rhythm are active participants. Because of the integration of many essential body functions in the CANS, and of the critical role of the heart in the maintenance of circulatory function, most homeostatic processes influence, and are influenced by, cardiac rhythm properties.

6.2 Heart Rate Definition Problems

One of the issues in HRV studies is the operational definition of the instantaneous HR, or the instantaneous HP. HR is conventionally given in beats per minute (bpm), a unit that evokes the image of the clinical behavior of sampling HR by actually counting the number of heart beats within a 1-minute interval. Clinicians often shorten the observation window from 60 seconds to 15 seconds and then multiply the counted beats by a factor of four to estimate the desired quantity, sacrificing precision for speed. Thus, the traditional clinical definition of HR is a count of events per unit time, with the events typically on the order of a second apart. A number of problems occur with defining instantaneous HR as a limiting condition of the traditional clinical concept. The idea of an instantaneous rate, continuously defined at every point in time, appears logically inconsistent. Even if definable, it remains essentially unknowable in the sense of being impossible to infer from measured data.

Figure 6.3–Development of HP sequence for use in HRV analyses: (a) Ideal atrial rate, (b) R-to-R interval, (c) A beat sequence vector (d) The beat lengths can be put in an appropriate but irregularly spaced placement in time, and interpolation of a continuous curve through these point may describe the unknowable instantaneous tendency of the heart period sequence, (e) An artificial HP sequence with uniform sampling.

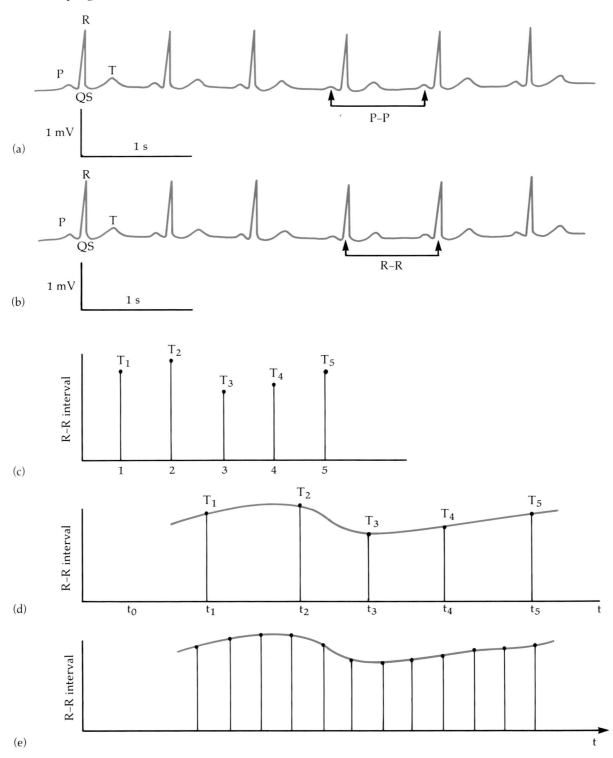

Practically, the instantaneous HR must be defined from a series of discrete events corresponding to the beating of the heart. This discrete event series itself is usually derived from fiducial features of the raw ECG waveform or pulse plethysmography local blood volume waveform. The former source provides a more detailed chronology of the microevents of the heart beat. The arrival time of a beat, and time interval from the last beat supply somewhat irregularly spaced information about short-term fluctuations in heart rhythm.

The use of HRV measures in research usually relates to theoretical models about autonomic control of the heart and its influence on the timing of the initiation of depolarization. Thus, most researchers base the definition of the interbeat interval (IBI) on the distance between adjacent P waves to reflect as closely as possible the statistics of the firing of the sinoatrial pacemaker node (Figure 6.3a). However, the P-to-P interval is much more difficult to empirically define than the R-to-R interval, particularly from noisy low-frequency Holter recordings of ambulatory subjects (Figure 6.3b). Most HRV studies, and essentially all those done using ambulatory ECG monitoring technology, employ the R-to-R interval as the fundamental metric.

The R-to-R intervals decoded from the actual ECG can be put into a beat length sequence in which the continuous length of each cardiac cycle is an interval measure, indexed by the integer beat sequence number. Each R-to-R interval can be inverted to a beat-specific equivalent HR, which can represent the equivalent rate that would have been observed if all the heart beats in a 60-second period had exactly that length. A beat-oriented data structure composed of a sequence of R-to-R intervals or instantaneous equivalent HRs is the fundamental unit of analysis for many common HRV summary statistics (Figure 6.3c).

The beats are not evenly spaced in time, however. If the analysis requires association with other real-time events in the body, such as respiration, the beat length vector may require an association with another vector to indicate exactly when in real-time each beat occurred. Philosophical problems arise in deciding whether the length of the beat is associated with the timing of the R wave that initiated the beat interval, or of the R wave that defined its end, or somewhere in between. The consequence of choosing the wrong end of the interval is an HR-dependent phase shift between the interval (rate) sequence and other real-time physiological states.

A continuous function can be defined at every point in time by interpolating a curve through the unevenly spaced set of (time, interval) ordered pairs corresponding to each beat. This function, while artificially constructed, satisfies some of the operational requirements for an instantaneous HP or HR signal (Figure 6.3d). The interpolated function can be as simple as a sample-and-hold in which the value of the previous interval is held constant until the next R wave arrives, creating an unlikely discontinuous stair-step approximation. This definition of the time function often is built into the electronic circuitry of biomedical instrumentation for the generation of a recordable analog output signal corresponding to HR. A linear interpolation between beats uses straight line segments to connect the irregularly spaced samples. But the slope or derivative of the function remains discontinuous at the points where the line segments intersect with different angles at the observed data values. Although many higher order polynomial and trigonometric interpolations exist, a number of HRV researchers employ cubic splices, the basis for the algorithms used by most computer graphics packages to draw visually pleasing smooth curves through data points. As discussed in a later section, evenly spaced time series of

HP (rate) data are commonly resampled from these interpolated curves to use the readily available time series modeling and spectral analysis software packages (Figure 6.3e).

6.3   *Which to Use: Heart Rate or Heart Period?*

One of the first decisions a researcher studying HRV must make is to select the fundamental unit of measurement: instantaneous HP or instantaneous HR. Both are reciprocally defined and carry the same theoretical information when used as instantaneous measures. But both can have very different statistical properties when aggregated within and across subjects. Instantaneous HP is commonly measured in milliseconds, or thousandths of a second, quantifying the temporal interval of the cardiac cycle. When derived from ECG signals, the period is noted as the duration between repetition of features in the ECG waveform, typically successive R waves. Instantaneous HR is measured in bpm and represents the equivalent bpm that would have been measured if that particular cardiac cycle rate had been maintained exactly throughout a full 60-second period.

The mathematical representation of the one-to-one relationship between these quantities is given by the equations:

$$HR(beats/min) = 60(sec/min) x \frac{1000(ms/sec)}{HP(ms/beat)}$$

Equation 6.1

$$HP(ms/beat) = 60(sec/min) x \frac{1000(ms/sec)}{HR(beats/min)}$$

Equation 6.2

While the relationship is a simple one, it is also *nonlinear*, which has stimulated a great deal of discussion about the relative merits of the two measures. From the one-to-one mapping through a slight nonlinearity, both measures carry the same information. However, at the level of practical science, some concerns about the distinctions exist. For example, if a researcher wishes to incorporate some measure of heart rhythm in a complex theoretical linear model with a number of other biopsychosocial dimensions, an overt assumption is that all the model variables must bear a linear relationship to each other. But if HR actually has linear relationships to the other variables in the model, then it is a mathematical tautology that HP cannot have linear relationships with the same variables. Similarly, if HP actually has a linear relationship to any study variable, then HR must have a nonlinear relationship with the same variable. This conclusion was noted by Graham and Jackson, who nevertheless remarked that the distortions introduced by the moderate nonlinearity may not be important in most applications.[105] However, Khachaturian and co-workers have suggested that using HR instead of HP in some applications may significantly distort relationships.[106] Similarly, Jennings, and colleagues have found that HP generally exhibits more linear behavior than HR.[107]

Measurement error becomes complex by the nonlinear relationship between period and rate. A uniform 1 bpm error corresponds to about a 24 ms error at 50 bpm, but only a 6 ms error at 100 bpm. Likewise a uniform 100 ms error is equivalent to a 5 to 7 bpm error at 1000 ms/beat, but a substantial 20 bpm error at 500 ms/beat. It is preferable to have the measurement error variance approximately homogeneous across the variations of heart rhythm that are likely to occur in the study under the set of clinical assessments.

Another issue closely related to linearity is the normality (Gaussianity) of the distributions of HR and HP representations of heart rhythm activity. A latent assumption of many classical statistical procedures is that the data are sufficiently normal and homogeneous in variance so that first and second order statistical moments (means, variances, and covariances) work. Once again, it is a mathematical tautology that if one of HR or HP is normally distributed, then the other cannot be because of the reciprocal nonlinearity between them. The relative degree of normality of HR and HP is very complex, and depends on whether the data is within-subject or within-group, whether multiple beats aggregate into a representative average or not, whether direct measures or lagged beat differences were collected, and whether neonates or adults were studied.[108,109] Within-subject data is often nonGaussian and nonhomogeneous for both HR and HP, but between-subject data is not. In adults, HP data has a somewhat more normal distribution, but HR presents a more Gaussian distribution for infants.

The previously cited studies contrasting HR and HP statistical properties were based on segments of data that were relatively short compared to that obtainable with modern ambulatory monitoring equipment. Twenty-four-hour HP and HR sequences both tend to be significantly nonnormal (nonGaussian). In fact, normal healthy subjects can produce heart rhythm distributions that are more statistically nonnormal than those recorded from cardiovascular patients. The major cause is circadian variation in HP and HR over 24-hour cycles. In Figure 6.4, the average hourly HP for a single subject is plotted from seven 24-hour recordings sampled over a period of 3 months. While unique variability exists in each 24-hour record, a strong day-night pattern occurs, with day-time average hourly peak rates reaching the equivalent of 100+ sustained bpm, and night-time average hourly rates dropping to about 60 bpm. At any moment in a pure circadian rhythm, a statistical tendency exists for the signal to be nearer one of the two extremes of the range than in the transition region in between. This results in a bimodal distribution with two maxima at the range extremes. In normal subjects, the circadian component may be the main source of general heart rhythm variability, with the CANS the primary mediating mechanism in its generation.

Meta-analysts trying to compare aggregated HP and/or HR measures across multiple studies often find major inconsistencies of 10% or more between averaged HR and HP data. The apparent paradox is that a between or within-subject average HR differs if computed by actually averaging instantaneous rate, or by averaging instantaneous HP and then inverting to an average rate measure. In the first approach, the average is computed with the equation:

$$\overline{HR_1} = \frac{1}{N}\sum_{j=1}^{N} HR_j \qquad \text{Equation 6.3}$$

and the second is effectively determined by:

$$\overline{HR_1} = \frac{1}{N}\sum_{j=1}^{N} HR_j \qquad \text{Equation 6.3}$$

A similar pair of equations can be written for the estimation of average HP. If the instantaneous period in the second equation is an inverse rate, it is apparent why the two estimates are different:

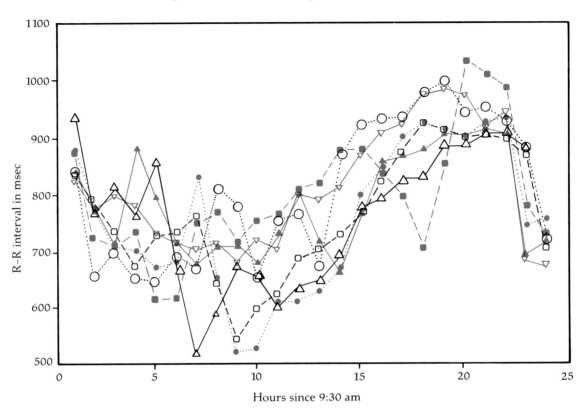

Figure 6.4–Superposition of seven 24-hour heart period records collected from a single subject over a 3-month period.

Figure 6.5–Cumulative survival after myocardial infarction for 808 subjects stratified into three groups on the basis of the Kleiger Global standard deviation heart rate variability measure.

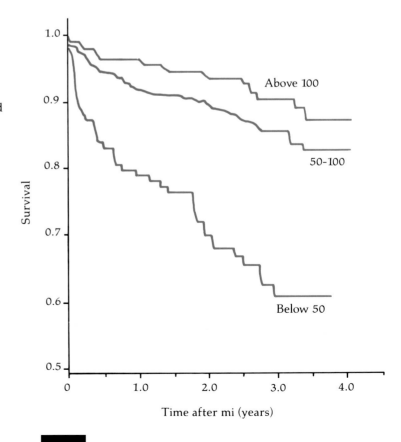

$$\overline{HR'_2} = \frac{60 \times 1000}{\dfrac{1}{N} \sum\limits_{J=1}^{N} \dfrac{60 \times 1000}{HR_J}}$$

Equation 6.5

Apart from the time conversion factors, which cancel out, this latter form is what is commonly called a *harmonic mean* of the rate, the inverse of the mean of inverses. The first method computes the more common *arithmetic mean*, which is known to be always larger than the harmonic mean except in the case when no variability exists in the data set. The simple nonlinear relation between *instantaneous* HR and HP does not hold between *averages* of HR and HP, even if the latter are computed over the identical set of data.

Higher order analyses such as standard deviations and spectra can be affected by the nonlinear definitional differences between the two descriptions of exactly the same underlying rhythm phenomenon. The decision to use HR or HP for the fundamental metric in a study is essentially nontechnical, and more a matter of convention and comparability with other researchers. The effect size of the study is likely to be so large that it overcomes any distributional peculiarities. The clinical interpretation is fairly comparable: having more than 10% variation over 24 hours of either HR or HP is generally a good sign, and having less than 5% variation in either HR or HP is probably not such a good sign. Most, but not all, heart rhythm studies currently analyze *HP variability*, but use the term *HR variability* in their title.

6.4 Time-Weighting Versus Beat-Weighting of Statistical Summaries

Another decision a clinician must make to initiate a project that includes HR information is whether to summarize the within-subject statistics on a beat- or a time-weighted basis. The distinction is largely philosophical, and the overall study effect size is not likely to be affected by the choice as long as it is consistently applied within the study. But large differences in the means and in the standard deviations of the two approaches are commonly observed. It is important to clearly indicate in reports and papers how the statistics were actually developed.

An example illustrating both philosophical and the computational issues is a 24-hour Holter ECG recording indicating that a subject had maintained an HP of 500 msec/beat (that is, an HR of 120 bpm) for the time interval from 9 AM to 9 PM, and then held a constant HP from 9 PM to 9 AM of 1000 msec/beat (60 bpm). The 24-hour mean HP calculated using beat weighing is 666.7 msec with a standard deviation of 240.3 msec. The 24-hour mean HP based on time weighing is 750 msec with a standard deviation of 257.1 msec. The difference reflects that during the first 12-hour period the heart was beating twice as fast and producing twice as many beats (86,400 beats) as it did during the second 12-hour period (43,200 beats). The beat-weighted estimate, which is simpler to compute, gives greater influence to periods with higher typical rate. A related effect that strongly influences the second order statistics but is not modeled by this simple artificial example is the observed tendency of short-term HP variation to be larger when the local average rate is slower (the HP longer). The beat-weighted quantification of the heart rhythm variability thus is often lower in amplitude than time-weighted estimates. The problem for the clinician is to decide which approach more appropriately characterizes the 24-hour heart rhythm behavior of the subject. The issue of beat time versus real time re-emerges in the context of time series methods and will be discussed in a later section.

6.5 *Heart Rate Variability Measures*

Most clinical and research applications of HRV measures are derived from 24-hour ambulatory monitoring. However, some HRV research is carried out using collected data segments that are much shorter, with almost every research paper seeming to use a different data collection interval. Unfortunately, the estimates of variation derived from a 30-second study cannot be directly compared with a 2-minute study, a 2-minute study with a 5-minute study, or an 8-hour study with a 24-hour study because the measured heart rhythm variation increases with increasing observation length. For longer segment analysis lengths (i.e., when comparing 1-hour and 6-hour HP sequences), more of the circadian variability falls within the analysis window. Only a few of the variability measures in use today have the same meaning when applied to segments of differing length (a potential exception is the root mean square of successive differences [RMSSD], defined below). Nevertheless, studies using standardized segment lengths from 30 seconds to several days have shown *within-study* consistency and valid effects in clinical comparisons. It is only in the extrapolation of the specific quantitative comparisons to broader domains that the limits of generalizability are reached.

A large number of convergent definitions exist for HRV based on 24-hour Holter ECG monitoring in the current literature. This diversity reflects the relative immaturity of rhythm variability analysis as an index of cardiac autonomic influences. The first three of the following measures are ad hoc summary statistics of 24-hour R-to-R interval sequences that make no explicit use of sequential dependencies or rhythmic behavior.

6.5.1 Kleiger Global Standard Deviation

The Kleiger Global Standard Deviation simply represents the beat-weighted standard deviation of the set of all the HPs (R-to-R intervals) in a 24-hour interval.[110] Kleiger and coworkers found this simple summary statistic was a powerful predictor of long-term mortality in acute myocardial infarction survivors (Figure 6.5). It conveyed independent information not captured by better-known clinical predictors.

6.5.2 Magid Statistic

The Magid Statistic is also known as the **AVESTD** and the **SDIndex**. It is the average of the standard deviations of successive 5-minute blocks over 24 hours.[111-113] The Magid measure is relatively sensitive to heart variation on a time scale less than 5 minutes, and is very insensitive to changes in average HR over time intervals longer than 5 minutes. It is a hybrid measure of beat and time weighing, with beat weighing of the SD within each 5-minute block, but an even weighing over the 24 hours for the mean of the 5-minute SDs. In measure evaluation studies at the University of Washington, the Magid SDIndex has generally performed no worse than other variability definitions in clinical contrasts, but seems to have unique properties of within-subject consistency. From collected multiple 24-hour tapes on individual subjects, this measure has demonstrated the greatest repeatability over time of any of the measures tested.

6.5.3   SDANN

SDANN is, in a sense, the complement of the Magid measure –the standard deviation of the means of successive 5-minute blocks over 24 hours.[114] The SDANN reflects heart variability on a time scale longer than 5 minutes and suppresses short-term heart rhythm fluctuations. The SDANN is the best indicator of the amplitude of circadian day/night variations in HR. It is also a hybrid beat- and time-weighted estimate, with beat weighing of the mean within each 5-minute block, yet uniform weighing over time in the determination of the SD of 5-minute means. While too diffuse a measure to assist in distinguishing the differential contributions of the sympathetic and parasympathetic branches of the CANS, the SDANN is consistently one of the best statistics for contrasting clinical cardiovascular conditions. The SDANN is also the most resistant against beat-labeling errors and movement artifact. For example, the occurrence of ectopic beats in a 5-minute analysis block has very little influence on the block average R-to-R interval length, especially if the nonsinus beats are classic PVCs with a short R-to-R interval followed immediately by a longer compensatory pause. The robustness of the SDANN can be further enhanced with little change in interpretation by substituting the median for the mean of each 5-minute block. The SDANN is the only variability measure discussed in this section that can be credibly estimated from the great variety of clinical equipment that performs running-average smoothing of the HR or HP sequence. Many manufacturers of clinical equipment designed to monitor heart rhythm over long time intervals have built in 3-beat, 5-beat, 7-beat, 21-beat, even 1-minute averagers to provide a more stable presentation of the main trends in the beat sequence. This attempt to filter out respiratory and other short-term sources of variation suppresses information essential to all of the HRV measures except SDANN. SDANN can be computed on any set of data that can reliably and consistently estimate an average HP for each 5-minute block throughout a full 24 hours.

As measures of simple process variability, the Kleiger Global SD, the Magid SD Index, and the SDANN do not distinguish if the interbeat intervals are totally random white noise or completely deterministic oscillations. Two well-known HRV measures use primitive information about the sequential properties of the HP data, focusing on the change in length of the current R-to-R interval from the immediately previous R-to-R interval. Significant changes on an instantaneous beat-to-beat basis are generally assumed to be precipitated by parasympathetic tone.

6.5.4   Ewing BB50, pNNSD, RMSSD

The Ewing BB50 statistic is the average over 24 hours of the number of occurrences per hour of the event that the difference between two successive R-to-R intervals exceeds 50 ms.[115] A near-variant, the **pNN50**, is the percent of absolute differences between successive normal beats that exceed 50 ms. Thus, the percentage-based pNN50 is normalized by the total number of R-to-R intervals in 24 hours (or equivalently the grand average HR), while the average hourly count-based BB50 is not normalized. The nature of the BB50 as a count of large rhythm changes makes it susceptible to outliers. Essentially every misclassified nonsinus beat contributes to the BB50 count.

The RMSSD is a measure of the variation of changes in R-to-R interval length from one beat to the next:

$$RMSSD = \sqrt{\frac{\sum_{i=1}^{n-1}(X_{i+1} - X_i)^2}{(n-1)}}$$

Equation 6.6

Based on beat-to-beat changes, the RMSSD is not sensitive to long-term drift and trend in the R-to-R interval sequence. Since the mean of first differences of a long-bounded sequence approaches zero, and as the standard deviation of a zero-mean sequence is mathematically equivalent to its root mean square, an excellent approximation to the RMSSD can be computed by determining the standard deviation of successive differences in common microcomputer or mainframe statistical packages without any special programming. The RMSSD is both insensitive to nonstationarities in the beat sequence and resistant against beat labeling errors and outliers.[116] Measure comparisons in our laboratory have confirmed that the RMSSD is largely insensitive to nonstationarities with a temporal scale longer than 10 seconds.[117] The RMSSD, like most methods based on sums of squares of observations, is not resistant to outliers such as improperly classified ectopic beats. However, slight changes in the RMSSD computation procedure to mitigate its dependence on extreme outliers, such as alpha-trimmed, winsorized, or bi-weight estimates, result in an exceptionally robust and resistant estimate of short-term variations in the heart rhythm sequence that may be a simple effective index of vagal influences.

Of all the measures tested, the RMSSD is the most invariant to the length of the observation interval. Thus, an RMSSD derived from a 5-minute sample is about the same expected magnitude as an RMSSD derived from a 24-hour sample, with several important qualifications. The sampling variability of the 5-minute segment is much greater than that of the 24-hour estimate. Also short- and long-term estimates of the RMSSD are greater if they span night-time hours because of circadian increases in fast variation of the heart rhythm during sleep.

An interesting measure that is not easily classified as a standard deviation, instantaneous change, or spectral frequency statistic is the heart rhythm spike count. Transient changes in rate with a magnitude of more than 10 equivalent bpm and a duration of 3 to 15 minutes are relatively frequent in normal patients but rare in cardiovascular patients.[117] When represented as a time series plot of heart rhythm expressed as rate and smoothed with a 1-minute rectangular moving average filter, spikes usually appear as upward-moving arousal events. When the rhythm data is plotted as the 1-minute average HP, the illustration resembles icicles hanging off the local baseline HP process. Spike events over 24-hour Holter tape records can be quantified as either a total count or a rate per hour. Seriously compromised patients often have five times fewer spike events per day than normal subjects.

Time series and power spectral analyses of the R-to-R interval sequence allow the fractionation of the effects of sympathetic and parasympathetic influences on the heart rhythm. These analyses are particularly effective for identifying and quantifying RSA. Many authors have discussed the efficacy of these models of the dynamic temporal dependencies of the R-to-R interval sequence.[118-122] Myers, for example, compared several of the previously described HRV measures with a spectral analysis approach, and found the spectral energy at respiratory and higher frequencies to be a powerful discriminator between groups of sudden cardiac arrest (SCA) patients, normal subjects, and nonSCA patients.[118]

A spectrum is a kind of histogram that measures the relative strength of rhythm patterns over a graded continuum of lengths. Fast rhythms map into peaks on the right of the spectrum, while slowly changing rhythms correspond to peaks on the left (Figure 6.6). When applied to HRV, mid-frequency peaks usually reflect parasympathetically-mediated RSA, and the low-frequency peaks indicate sympathetic and reciprocal sympathetic-parasympathetic reflex activity. The sympathetic nervous system appears responsive only at frequencies below approximately 0.1 Hz (rhythm patterns 10 seconds or longer), while the parasympathetic nervous system can mediate much faster rhythmic processes.[123] Figure 6.7 shows three segments of real HP sequence data illustrating common rhythm patterns and their corresponding spectra.

In the previous examples, the spectrum qualitatively depicted the distribution of rhythm patterns in the data sequence, but visual observation of the time domain data could have led to the same general conclusions. Spectral HRV analysis often provides very unique insight into complex heart rhythm properties. The HP series and spectrum are presented for a subject in two postural states: standing and supine (Figure 6.8).[118] Comparison of the two spectra allows interpretation of the effects of postural adjustment that would have been difficult to infer from observation of the corresponding time series.

Four main approaches are used for the spectral analysis of heart rhythm sequences. Both nonparametric and parametric spectral methods can be applied to HP sequences that are indexed either by beat number or real time. The four possibilities thus generated are frequently seen in the HRV analysis literature.

6.5.5   Frequency Versus Beatquency

The HP interbeat interval sequence is composed of R-to-R intervals decoded from the raw ECG, indexed by the integer beat sequence number, and possibly augmented by an additional vector coding the placement in real consecutive time of each beat. The beat information is not evenly spaced in time, but some authors choose to compute a spectrum over the nonuniform time base of the beat index itself, which is often called "beat time" or "metabolic time" to distinguish it from "real time." The resulting HRV spectrum has an abscissa called the "beatquency" with units in *cycles per beat* to distinguish it from the real-time equivalent frequency axis and its units of *cycles per second*. The convention for presentation of these spectra labels the x-axis with two scales: the first as *beatquency* (cycles per beat) and the second as *equivalent frequency*, computed by dividing the beatquency by the average R-to-R interval for that analysis block (Figure 6.9).

Other researchers prefer to decompose the spectral structure with respect to a real-time base. A continuous function can be defined at every point in time by interpolating a curve through the unevenly spaced set of ordered pairs (time, interval) corresponding to each beat. Cubic spline interpolation usually works well for HRV data, with practical software easily obtained. Evenly spaced time series of HP (rate) data are commonly resampled from these interpolated curves to apply commonly available time series modeling and spectral analysis software packages. The resampling rate is often several times faster than the natural HR: in adults two or four times per second, in infants four or eight times per second. The resulting sequence has natural time units, and the corresponding spectrum has the usual frequency interpretation, with units in cycles per second.

Because it avoids the interpolation step, the beatquency approach is easier to implement. For short stationary segments of data, it produces excellent spectra that describe the major features of interest, especially the low and high frequency peaks. Because of the beat-by-beat distortions in its time base, the HRV beatquency spectrum has a weaker functional connection to external real-time processes such as respiration. It is difficult to

Figure 6.6–The amplitude of the rhythm determines the height of the spectral peak, here plotted on the logarithmic dB scale.

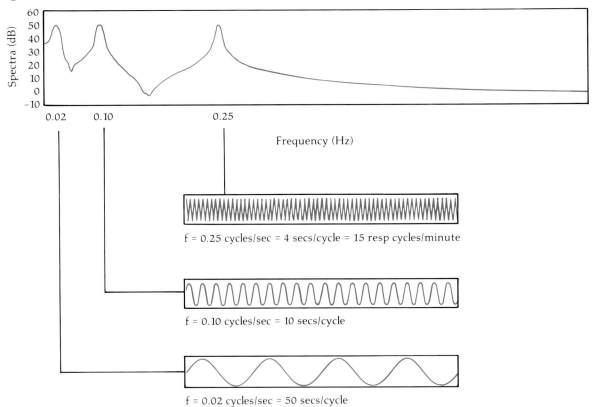

f = 0.25 cycles/sec = 4 secs/cycle = 15 resp cycles/minute

f = 0.10 cycles/sec = 10 secs/cycle

f = 0.02 cycles/sec = 50 secs/cycle

Figure 6.7–Representative segments of actual HP sequence data, illustrating typical rhythmic patterns and the corresponding spectral representations. (a) 500-second segment of HP data. (b) 100-second segment of HP data. (c) A segment of HP data from the same subject with a strong RSA component having a period of about 5 seconds.

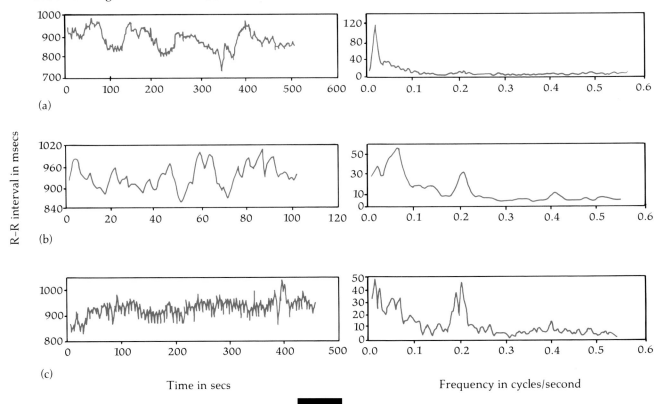

(a)

(b)

(c)

R-R interval in msecs

Time in secs

Frequency in cycles/second

average over segments with varying average HP. Spectra, based on sequences interpolated into real time, preserve the natural temporal mapping to other real-time processes in the body and are easily averaged. However, the interpolation approximates an unknowable continuous sinus drive function. The consequences of synthesizing data by approximation and resampling are difficult to assess.

6.5.6 Traditional Versus Autoregressive Model-Based Spectral Analysis

Many of the applications of HRV spectral analysis employ the traditional Discrete-Fourier transform (DFT) of either the HP sequence or an estimate of its autocovariance function. Implementations for large amounts of data, such as those collected on 24-hour Holter ambulatory monitors, can result with the very efficient Fast-Fourier transform (FFT) algorithm of the DFT procedure. The data sequences divide into 1-to-5 minute segments, each of which has about the same spectral properties. The block spectra can then be averaged into hourly spectra, or even a representative 24-hour spectrum. The DFT-based spectra are subject to a very serious artifact called "sidelobes" due to the finite length of the data sequence. Sidelobes spread information about spectral peaks inappropriately throughout the frequency band. The sidelobes can make it appear that substantial activity exists at both low and high frequencies when the activity only occurs at low frequencies.

Sidelobes can be reduced by tapering the data sequence with multiplicative bell-shaped "windows", and essentially giving more weight to the data in the middle, but almost no weight to the data near the edges of the analysis block. While this manipulation protects against sidelobes, it reduces the effective number of degrees of freedom in the analysis block because the data near the edges are essentially discarded. Overlapping the data blocks by 50% fully exploits the information in the data sequence. A comprehensive review of the use of windows in DFT/FFT procedures has been developed.[124]

Even when all the data degrees of freedom are retained, the DFT/FFT periodogram for each analysis block is statistically very unstable. Each point in the raw DFT/FFT periodogram estimate of the spectrum effectively represents only two independent data degrees of freedom. The spectrum represents a kind of model of the data that include just twice as many data points (the input data sequence) as there are parameters (the estimated points on the DFT/FFT periodogram curve). A great deal of the data sequence randomness passes onto the parameters, which will have the equivalent statistical stability of the mean of two random numbers. The process of windowing to control sidelobes further reduces the statistical reliability of a raw periodogram of a single block of HP data. The random variance of the spectral estimates can be significantly decreased by averaging sets of adjacent DFT/FFT frequency bins together. However, this smears spectral features, broadening peaks and generally reducing the frequency resolution of the estimate. Bendat and Piersol discuss the practical tradeoffs between stationarity, sidelobe leakage, statistical stability, and frequency resolution.[125]

Parametric autoregressive model-based spectral analysis can be applied to HP sequences as an alternative to traditional nonparametric (hyperparametric) DFT/FFT approaches. The method is based on the tautology that, for every autoregressive time series model, an equivalent spectrum exists. Thus, parameters for an autoregressive model can be estimated from a block of data, then interpreted as a spectrum. Some advantages of the autoregressive model-based spectrum include no sidelobes, greater statistical stability,

Figure 6.8–The visual difference between the HP sequences of a subject in two postural states is somewhat subtle. However spectral analysis reveals dramatically different dynamic properties in the two records.

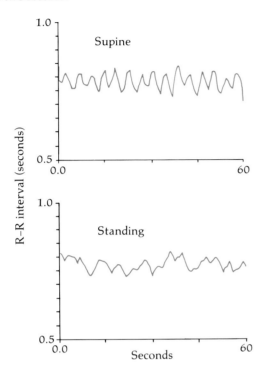

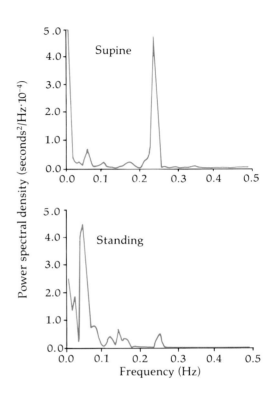

Figure 6.9–Examples of spectra computed with respect to cycles/beat rather than cycles/second.

(a)

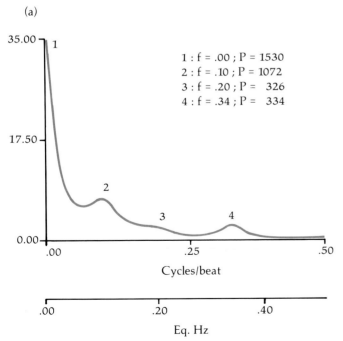

1 : f = .00 ; P = 1530
2 : f = .10 ; P = 1072
3 : f = .20 ; P = 326
4 : f = .34 ; P = 334

(b)

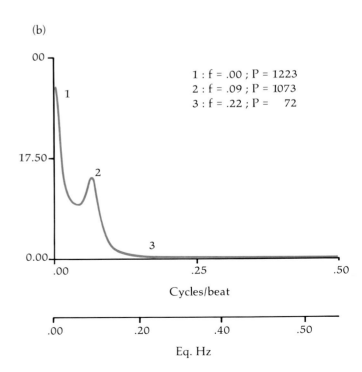

1 : f = .00 ; P = 1223
2 : f = .09 ; P = 1073
3 : f = .22 ; P =   72

and excellent resolution of sharp peaks. The statistical stability results from the relatively small number of autoregressive parameters that describe an HRV spectrum. The laboratory experience shows that an autoregressive model with a parametric order between 10 and 25 (typically 15) does an excellent job of specifying the spectrum of an 512-point HP sequence.[126] The ratio of data points to parameters is thus much higher (~20:1 to 50:1) than that of the traditional DFT/FFT (~2:1).

Autoregressive methods work well in analysis situations requiring very sharp resolution of a small number of peaks, which is exactly what occurs in HRV analyses. The technique does not generally require any tapering windows in the time domain or smoothing windows in the frequency domain. However, an appropriate order for the analysis model must be determined, and is the key determinant of the quality of the resulting spectral estimate. If the model order is too low, the spectrum becomes too simple and smooth. If the model order is too high, the spectrum contains unrealistic and statistically unreproducible detail. The autoregressive model-based spectra are computationally much less efficient than FFT-based traditional approaches, which have inexpensive hardware for extremely fast performance.

An example of traditional nonparametric spectral analysis applied to beat time HP sequences is presented by Lisenby and Richardson.[127] Autoregressive spectral models of beat time HP sequences and their application are carefully developed by Baselli and co-workers.[126] Myers and co-workers have presented the classic treatment of nonparametric spectral analysis to HP sequences interpolated into real time.[118] The autoregressive spectra computed from interpolated real-time HP sequences are employed in many HRV analyses.[128] With some care, each of these four basic approaches can be used to develop interpretable spectra as a part of HRV studies.

Spectral analysis add to HRV studies because mid-frequency peaks can usually be interpreted as having a respiratory origin and parasympathetic mediation. For any given HRV spectrum, this is guesswork, based on reasonable principles, but unsupported by any specific evidence except that the rhythmic patterns in the HP sequence have periods about the same length as typical respiration cycle periods. If respiration can be simultaneously measured, multivariate spectral analysis can largely remove the ambiguity of the connection between specific respiratory pattern events and changes in HP sequences. In addition to computing the usual spectra for both respiration and HP, multivariate spectral analysis develops a cross-spectral description of a linear model between the two series. The coherence spectrum depicts the R^2 of the best linear model of the variations in the HP data at each frequency in terms of the variations in the respiratory behavior at exactly the same frequency. A mid-band peak in the coherence spectrum is extremely strong evidence that a peak at the same frequency in the HP autospectrum actually quantifies RSA. A coherence-weighted spectrum is a variant of the typical HRV spectrum that factors in the confirmability of the association with respiration. In addition to describing the frequency-specific strength of coupling between respiration and HP, multivariate spectral analysis can determine the phase spectrum, measuring a frequency-specific time delay between cause (respiration) and effect (HP variation). Any researcher collecting HP data in the laboratory should probably simultaneously sample some estimate of the raw respiratory waveform if logistically possible because of the tremendous increase in strength of the inferences about RSA. The next generation of 24-hour ambulatory Holter recorders are being developed to simultaneously measure respiratory excursions.

The spectra computed for blocks of HP sequences throughout the 24-hour Holter collection period can be averaged into a grand mean spectrum. While this summary plot de-

Figure 6.10–Perspective plot of 24-hour HRV spectra.

HRV	Acute MI	6 Month follow-up
Kleiger	65.4 msec	93.5 msec
Magid	34 msec	38 msec
SDANN	56 msec	85 msec
BB50	217 occ/hour	311 occ/hour

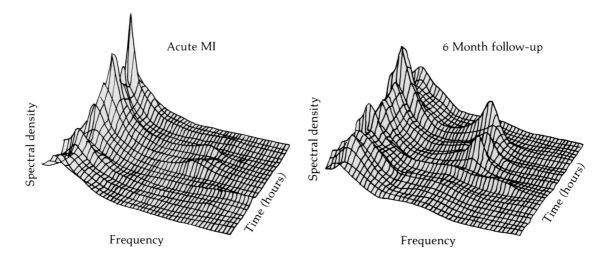

Figure 6.11–Respiratory rates less than six breaths per minute can result in RSA patterns that masquerade as Mayer waves.

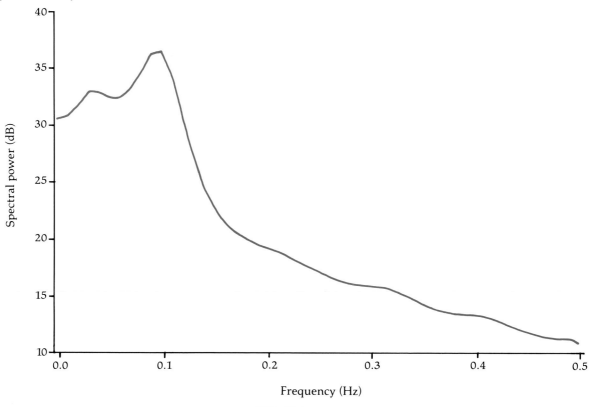

scribes the typical relative concentrations of variations at various frequencies, it does not do justice to the modulation over time of the relative preponderance of long slow rhythms over short fast rhythms or vice versa. This meta-variability in spectral distribution reflects the rapidly changing contributions of the theoretical CANS subcomponents. At every time scale capable of resolution, changes occur.

Several graphics allow us to understand the variation of spectral energy over time. For example, Figure 6.10 presents a perspective plot of the hourly spectral distribution through 24 hours in a normal subject. The mid-frequency peaks representing the theoretically important RSA primarily occur during sleep in the subject's 24-hour day. The contour plot offers a comparable form of display for time varying spectral information. When the desired time resolution is acceptable, but the total recording interval is long, the perspective and contour plots become somewhat unwieldy. Compressed spectral arrays and top-down gray scale displays, long employed for spectral analyses of time-varying electroencephalography, speech, and radar signals, allow very compact depiction of the redistributions of HRV spectral energy.

Summarizing the points from the above description and examples of HRV spectra: over a 24-hour perspective, the HP time series is not stationary; interpretation is usually limited to extraction of the amount of variation or energy falling in a small number of bands each having fairly well-understood frequency boundaries; and in normal subjects at least, the energy distribution in the bands can change very rapidly. Many applications do not require formal computation of a spectrum to understand the relative balance of slow rhythms and fast rhythms. A digital filter system for partitioning the slow and fast components, then measuring the strength of these separate variations, can be specified in a software analysis program analogous to a hardware filter bank in analog instrumentation. Because the amount of variation in a band can be rapidly estimated from a relatively small section of data using this approach, markers for the sympathetic and parasympathetic tone can dynamically track the modulation of the CANS with a time resolution much less than a minute. For example, Shin, and colleagues demonstrated the changes in HRV rhythm properties in a dog expecting to be shocked in a conditioned stimuli experiment to a 5-second resolution using complex demodulation, a time series approach closely related to spectral analysis.[122]

Nonlinear dynamic systems analysis techniques, including chaos theory approaches, are being applied to HP data sets.[129] HP sequences collected from normal subjects appear chaotic to some observers. Several aspects of the heart rhythm support this view. HP data visually appears to have fluctuations of the same structure when plotted on many different time scales, a property of self-similarity essential to the definition of a fractal. The trajectory of many chaotic processes is confined to a fractal object in state-space. With the exception of a few major features like the respiration-induced mid-frequency RSA peak, the HRV spectrum approximates a 1/f distribution, again consistent with the HP sequence being the outcome of a chaotic system. Some evidence of subharmonic bifurcations in rate results in congestive heart failure patients, demonstrating an extreme sensitivity to initial conditions and perturbations diagnostic of chaotic generating mechanisms.[130] Finally, anyone who has been trained in nonlinear dynamics can see structures in the low-frequency oscillations of the HP sequence that resemble the outputs of simple nonlinear differential equations. It is widely accepted that the HP sequence in healthy persons and in those with cardiovascular illness results from an aggregation of a large number of sometimes strongly nonlinear inputs. Thus, nonlinear dynamic system analysis approaches can be very informative.

The claim that the HP series is fundamentally chaotic remains controversial, however, because dynamic systems can be nonlinear without being chaotic. The evidence of chaotic behavior presented to date, while probably proving that nonlinear mechanisms apply here, is consistent with the existence of an underlying chaotic system.

At present, the field of nonlinear dynamics is supported by elegant analytic results and a powerful simulation science, but plagued by poorly developed empirical methodologies. Given a real biological time series, there is nothing comparable to the various methods for inferring model structure, model order, and parameter estimates available for the linear case. The state of the science is to estimate the *complexity* of the hypothetical underlying nonlinear generating system, where the complexity plays a role similar to that of the model order. Only rarely are structural or parameter estimation inferences attempted, and then only under conditions of significant prior knowledge.

The complexity property of nonlinear generating system can be empirically quantified in several ways. Lyapunov exponents, estimates of the sensitivity of the system to initial conditions and perturbations, are exceptionally difficult to estimate directly from HP time series. Most nonlinear HRV analysts attempt to approximate the fractal or Hausdorff dimension.[131] This number is perhaps an estimate of the number of independent nonlinear oscillating subsystems contributing to the observed HP signal. If Hausdorff dimension is not an integer, for example 5.27, then a strong possibility exists that the underlying system is chaotic. Three basic algorithms to approximate the fractal dimension can be found in the HRV literature: the Box-Counting Algorithm, the Grassberger-Proccacia Algorithm, and the Takens-Ellner Algorithm. These methods are computationally intensive, often taking 24 hours to complete a computation on an hour's worth of HP data when run on a PC-386 computer. Details on their implementation can be found in basic references on the application of empirical nonlinear time series techniques.[132-138]

The nominal estimates of the Hausdorff dimension reported in the literature have had a rough positive association with simple variance estimates of HRV. For example, Mayer-Kress and colleagues report fractal dimensions d = 4.8 + 1.9 for HP segments taken during the day when HRV estimates are typically low, and d > 7.0 for HP segments taken during the night when HRV estimates are typically high.[139] The exact role that nonlinear dynamic analysis techniques, in particular generalized dimension and other systemic complexity estimates, will play in understanding HP sequences of normal subjects and cardiovascular patients is not clear at the present time. Chaos theory has given us the new perspective on biological time series that variation can arise from sources other than randomness or sinusoidal oscillations. Chaotic variation can appear quite random, yet may originate in completely deterministic nonlinear mechanisms.

6.6   *Identification of Nonsinus Beats*

Even in normal subjects, not all heart beats originate in the sinoatrial node. Premature and other nonsinus beats may represent a significant fraction of a cardiovascular patient's total number of beats in a 24-hour window. Nonsinus beats do not directly reflect the mediating influence of the CANS, although the amount of sympathetic and parasympathetic tone does indirectly affect the probability of production of ectopic beats. Since the purpose of most HRV studies is to elucidate the CANS, nonsinus beats contribute only noise to the estimates of system variation. Because the R-to-R intervals of premature and other nonsinus beats can differ from their neighbors, they contribute large amounts of unrelated variance to traditional nonresistant statistical measures of spread such as standard deviation.

Normal beats immediately following a nonsinus beat may be strongly influenced by the rhythm disturbance, both because of direct phase resetting and baroreflex control system adjustments. Compensations in R-to-R interval values must be observed for at least 10 seconds after a nonsinus event, although most effects have been damped out within three beats. For the common class of ectopic beat known as the premature ventricular contraction (PVC), the short R-to-R interval terminates with the arrival of the premature nonsinus beat and is followed by a compensatory long R-to-R interval that, in most cases, nearly corrects for the phase distortion in beat timing. Segments in the data affected by movement artifact also do not reliably communicate information about the CANS-mediated inputs to the sinus node. In 24-hour Holter ambulatory tapes, short sections of movement artifact are fairly common. Given that nonsinus beats and movement artifact do not reliably reflect CANS status, it remains difficult to identify and label beats and segments that are not useful and to condition the statistical analyses so that nonsinus beats do not bias the HRV summary statistics.

Beat status can be determined by direct observation of the raw ECG by an experienced ECG analyst, but to achieve anywhere near 100% accuracy on a 24-hour Holter tape requires a tremendous amount of effort. Many HRV analysis projects infer nonsinus beats not from the raw ECG, but from sudden changes in the HP sequence. This kind of rule misses ectopic beats falling within the percent change window, and discards information-rich normal intervals showing great change from one beat to the next. The best approach, when possible, is to use a modern Holter analysis system with both morphological and premature beat analysis capacity.

As noted earlier, the rhythm of a number of the normal beats following an ectopic beat can exhibit large transients that have the potential to make large contributions to the estimate of the intrinsic HRV. Most HRV analysts consider these succeeding 3 to 10 beats to be abnormal in the sense of not typical of the unperturbed heart rhythm response. They then flag them as not directly relevant to normal HRV. Some sensitivity studies have found no benefit to labeling more than the first three postectopic beats as abnormal. Indeed, there seems to be very little advantage to labeling more than one postectopic beat, but labeling the very next beat does make a significant difference. The perturbation in postectopic normal beats is itself mediated by the CANS and, in its own way, constitutes information about CANS functional capacities. It should also be noted that succeeding beats do not need to be flagged following movement artifact segments. Movement artifact represents an aberration of the monitoring capacity, not a perturbation of the real signal.

Most HRV analysis procedures cope with nonsinus beats and movement artifact segments by deletion beats flagged as abnormal are removed from the analysis. Many modern statistical procedures also allow selective weighting of data. Abnormal R-to-R intervals could be adaptively deweighted in the analysis to minimize estimate bias.

Nonapplicable and missing data segments create special problems for time-series and spectral analysis approaches to HRV studies. Commonly available software usually assumes that the data is in the form of a fairly lengthy sequence containing no missing data. The implications of this assumption will be discussed in a later section on special considerations for the use of HRV methods in clinical research designs.

Figure 6.12–Three cases studies contrasting HRV spectra during REM (Color) and non-REM sleep.

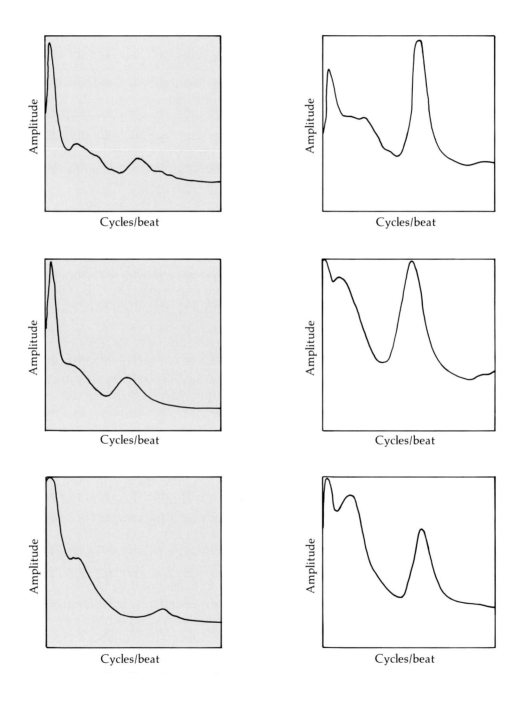

6.7   *Heart Rate Variability as a Measure in Clinical Environment*

When HRV measures are used in clinical practice, several methodological issues naturally arise all essentially concerned with whether observed qualities of the heart rhythm can be uniquely ascribed to alternations of tone in the CANS. This section discusses threats to the validity of simple interpretations of HRV measures from the perspective of clinical practice. For example, Figure 6.10 describes several HRV measures in a typical AMI survivor making a good recovery, constrasting CANS indicators shortly after the AMI event with those measured 6 months later.

Most HRV measures appear to suffer from the "passive observation problem" for a state variable in a complex system. The magnitude of the observed fluctuations depends on system dynamic response to uncontrolled internal and external stimuli. The observed variation may represent only a lower bound to that which is possible for the system. If the stimuli environment is systematically different at each longitudinal measurement wave, then observed changes in HRV may not just be due to alterations in the mediating CANS. In a longitudinal study of recovery after AMI, for example, the demands for somatic and psychologic activity can be much greater at a 6-month follow-up visit than during the hospitalization phase, with possible consequences for the interpretability of the HRV measures. More active patients produced slightly more long-term HRV, but slightly less short-term HRV.

The extraction of an index of parasympathetic tone from the RSA peak in the HRV spectrum is usually done by measuring the height of the peak at a particular frequency or the area under the curve in a prespecified band. If sufficient parasympathetic tone exists, the configuration of the RSA peak is driven by respiratory behavior: respiration at a regular rate produces a tall thin peak, while respiration at an irregular rate produces a low broad hill. Thus, peak height measures are presumed sensitive to the stability of the respiratory rate as well as to the level of parasympathetic tone. The summated spectral density in a band can be more comparable in these cases, but it is difficult to specify credible band boundaries. Sustained respiratory rates as low as six breaths per minute, which is manifested as a RSA peak in the spectrum at 0.1 Hz, have been observed (Figure 6.11).[40] This is well below the various RSA bands proposed in the literature. Such a peak would probably be misidentified as Mayer wave baroreflex oscillations and be given a very different ANS interpretation. More generally, some structural changes in the HRV spectra simply reflect changes in respiratory behavior.

The decision about discarding data from the analysis is always difficult. The proportion of the record affected by nonsinus and movement artifact segments is very likely conditioned by clinical status. HR data is very nonstationary at several time scales, with large changes in rhythm structure perhaps related to circadian rhythm, stage of sleep, and other more phasic factors. Common practices of selecting the "cleanest" or "most stationary" subsets of the data could lead to unconscious bias and manipulation. Some subjects may have essentially no qualifying data under the most stringent exclusion rules.

Posture has a profound effect on the rhythm structure of the HR signal, as evidenced in the HRV spectra (Figure 6.8). The RSA-induced spectral peak, which often occurs when the subject lies down, is reduced by an order of magnitude when the subject stands. An evaluative problem results if the patient spends a different percentage of time in postures than normal. For example, AMI patients spend a greater amount of time lying down in the hospital phase than they do 6 months later when most have resumed regular daily activities.

During normal sleep, the largest amount of HRV is generally measured. But even during sleep, large changes occur in the presentation of the HRV. A significant shift in the HRV spectrum is associated with discharges during rapid eye movement (REM) sleep (Figure 6.12). Marked decreases in the parasympathetically mediated mid-frequency bands appear. Thus, a randomly chosen section of heart rhythm data, even one sampled during sleep, may give an unrepresentative view of the subject's capacity to modulate sympathovagal tone. If the contrasts in the research design vary in the amount or timing of REM, differences in HRV summary statistics may be observed.

The CANS is strongly influenced by psychological happenings and psychosocial context, and plays a key role in the generation and perception of emotional responses. Even mild cognitive psychological stressors such as checkbook balancing arithmetic tasks and anagram "word jumble" tasks routinely cause phasic changes in the HRV as large as any physiological manipulation. After a very short reactive transient, HRV is much reduced after cognitive loading or affective experience, consistent with a model of sympathetic activation and vagal withdrawal.

For real clinical populations, the effects of drugs on HRV must be considered. Many medications prescribed for cardiovascular populations are specifically designed to modify heart rhythm and to affect the balance of the central ANS. Changes in the HRV spectrum related to beta-blocker and calcium channel blocker formulations have been demonstrated and enhancement of the spectral peak associated with RSA in patients receiving the vagomimetic scopolamine has been observed.[140,141]

The sensitivity and generality of HRV effects raise methodological issues for both longitudinal and independent groups research designs in clinical settings. It is also important to remember that the HRV statistics provide an accurate picture of the CANS under the observed conditions. It is the CANS that is subject to the limits of methodology, with the HRV measures merely reflecting alterations of CANS activity. Multiple factors can induce changes in the CANS, and hence in the HRV. Nevertheless, HR variability offers sensitive systemic measure that has demonstrated both practical utility and theoretical relevance for clinicians and researchers alike.

7.0 LATE POTENTIALS AND THE ELECTROCARDIOGRAM

The conventional electrocardiogram (ECG) consists of the P wave, QRS complex, T wave, and associated intervals (Figure 2.1). The P wave represents atrial depolarization, the QRS ventricular depolarization, and the T wave ventricular phase 4 repolarization. The ST segment records early ventricular repolarization. The standard ECG is read from ECG strip-chart paper (Figure 2.1). A fixed scale of 25 mm per second in the x direction and 100 µV per mm in the y direction is customarily used. The resolution of this printout is limited primarily by the sensitivity of the recording, and is further limited by the accuracy of the plotting device, pen width, and other factors. In consequence, ECG signals below 50 µV in amplitude and of less than 10 msec duration are not observed in the conventional ECG.

The first high-resolution ECG recordings were produced in the 1970s.[142] These studies focused on ECG signals representing the specialized conducting system.[143] Small signals — in the range of 0.5 to 10 µV — where found in the PR interval which previously had been considered an isoelectric interval. More recently, ventricular late potentials have become the primary application of the high-resolution ECG. Late potentials are low-level signals within the heart that arise from slow or delayed conduction in the border zone of a myocardial infarction.[144] They are linked to the presence of a re-entry substrate for ventricular tachycardia. The high-resolution ECG has become a useful noninvasive test for identifying patients at high risk for ventricular tachycardia. Late potentials, which can range from 1 to 20 µV, are below the resolution of standard ECG equipment.

Figure 7.1 shows late potentials in the high-resolution ECG. This illustration demonstrates some points that differ between the standard and high-resolution ECGs. Figure 7.1a shows the high-resolution ECG on more conventional time and amplitude scales. Figure 7.1b shows the same tracing at 10x the amplitude scale. The ECG appears normal except for the late QRS deflection, labeled LP.

Three essential differences exist between standard and high-resolution ECGs. The high-resolution ECG preserves low-level signals on the order of microvolts, which are usually not seen in an individual beat since they are masked by noise. The technique of signal averaging has been widely used to recover high-resolution ECG signals. Some separation of high-resolution ECG signals from the familiar normal QRS and ST segment waveforms must occur before interpretation. This has been accomplished by filtering and spectral analysis. The display of high-resolution ECG data is flexible. Different time and amplitude scales and aspect ratios (the ratio of the amplitude and time intervals or proportion of the ECG tracing) are easily achieved due to computerization of the procedure. These issues will be considered further in the presentation of signal averaging methods that follows.

7.1 *Recording the High-Resolution Electrocardiogram*

Recording of the high-resolution ECG is a computer-controlled process. It consists of four stages: ECG registration at the body surface, amplification and filtering, sampling, and patient isolation. Figure 7.2 presents a schematic of modern high-resolution ECG instrumentation.

Figure 7.1–The high-resolution ECG.

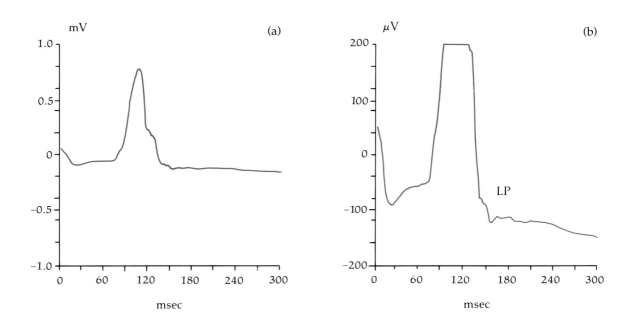

Figure 7.2–Overview of a high-resolution ECG system.

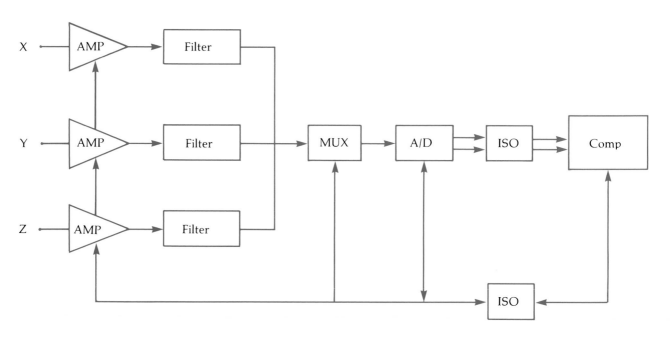

7.1.1   Registration

Typically, three orthogonal XYZ leads are used to record the high-resolution ECG. Proper application of the electrodes is an important step in quality control of the high-resolution ECG. The skin should be well braided and silver/silver chloride electrodes applied, ideally a few minutes in advance of recording to allow the electrical characteristics of the skin-electrode interface to stabilize. Problems with excessive noise in the high-resolution ECG often result from inadequate skin preparation and electrode application. The three bipolar, orthogonal lead sites are as follows: On the left midclavicular line, the negative and positive Y electrodes lie in the subclavicular space and the lower thoracic quadrant, respectively. The anteroposterior line defines the Z axis. The positive Z electrode is placed anteriorly on the Y axis at the fourth intercostal place. The negative Z electrode is placed correspondingly on the back. The positive and negative X electrodes are placed at the left and right midaxillary lines, respectively.[145]

7.1.2   Amplification and Filtering

From the electrodes, the transduced ECG signal is amplified and filtered (Figure 7.2). The amplification gain may be computer-programmable and set by the user (Figure 7.2). The amplifiers should be low noise and should exhibit high rejection of 60Hz interference. ECG instrumentation design involves many considerations and several good references are available.[146]

Electronic filtration of the signal serves two purposes: Highpass filtering at 0.05 Hz controls baseline wander and removes DC potentials. Lowpass filtering at 300 Hz attenuates noise outside the frequency range of the ECG signal. It also prevents aliasing, a problem related to sampling whereby high frequency noise can distort the lower-frequency ECG signal. For the high-resolution ECG, signals in the frequency band of 0.05 to 300 Hz are preserved. This is in contrast to the American Heart Association (AHA) specification of 0.05 to 100 Hz for the conventional ECG. The most advanced high-resolution ECG instrumentation contains no highpass filtering, passing all frequencies from 0 to 300 Hz. A seemingly small modification, it introduces both a major advantage and a significant difficulty. DC coupling means that no filter-induced phase shifts or distortions are introduced in the ST segment or QRS. This type of distortion has been a very significant problem, particularly with the ambulatory ECG.[147] However, DC potentials and ECG baseline wander must now be contained without filtering.

7.1.3   Sampling

Before digital sampling, the three simultaneous XYZ analog signals were multiplexed (operation "MUX" in Figure 7.2). In this operation, each signal is presented in turn to the A/D converter and is digitized. The digital value is then read into computer memory. This procedure takes only a few µsecs. The high-resolution ECG is typically sampled at a rate of 1,000 to 2,000 samples per second. The interval between sampling is 1 or 0.5 msec, respectively. At each sampling instant, every 500 µsec, all three leads are sampled in turn in typically 10 to 50 µsecs. Sampling of the three leads is therefore approximately simultaneous and easily accomplished before the next sample is due. The switching of the multiplexer and the operation of the A/D converter are synchronized by the computer (labeled "COMP" in Figure 7.2).

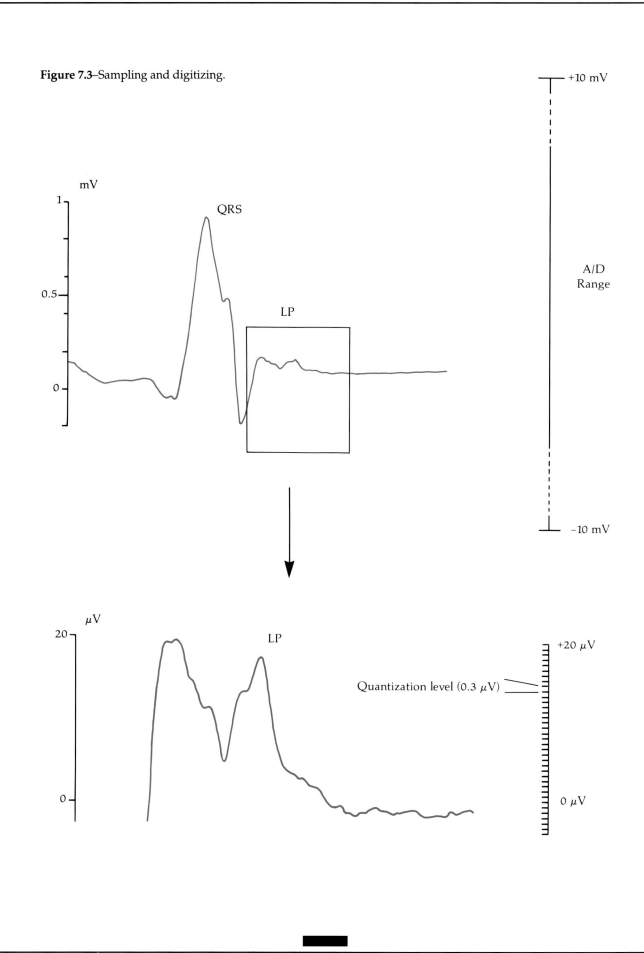

Figure 7.3–Sampling and digitizing.

Figure 7.3 graphically analyzes the sampling process. The ECG typically ranges from 1 to 3 mV, so the voltage range of the A/D converter must accommodate both the ECG signal and any DC potentials or baseline wander that may be present. The A/D range in this example is ±10 mV (Figure 7.3a). Figure 7.3b shows a blow-up of the 20 μV late potential signal. At each sampling instant, the ECG signal is quantized. The A/D converter selects the nearest quantization level to the ECG signal value. The number of quantization levels present is specified by the number of bits of the A/D converter. A 12-bit A/D converter can represent 4096 (2^{12}) values, and a 16-bit converter 65536 (2^{16}) values.

The resolution or quantization step of the A/D converter is determined by both its voltage range and number of bits (Figure 7.3). For example, a ±10 mV, 16-bit A/D converter has a resolution of 20 mV/65536 ≈ 0.3 μV. By comparison a similar 12-bit A/D converter has a resolution of only 20 mV/4096 ≈ 4.9 μV. A larger voltage range reduces resolution but is desirable, with DC-coupled instrumentation to accommodate baseline wander. A/D converters with more than 16 bits are costly and sometime less accurate, so a compromise resolution of 2.5 μV maximum is appropriate. The error between the true value of the signal and the nearest quantization level is known as quantization noise. This particular form of noise is reduced by the signal averaging technique described below.

7.1.4 Isolation

The instrumentation connected to the patient must be electrically isolated from the main electrical supply. This is achieved by inserting isolation circuitry into the signal path (labeled "ISO" in Figure 7.2). All instrumentation to the left of this circuitry must either be battery powered or have an electrically isolated power supply. The control signals from the computer to the amplifiers, multiplexer, and A/D converter must also be isolated (Figure 7.2). Isolation is achieved using either optical, magnetic, or capacitative coupling devices. Isolation of the digital signal is preferred since analog isolation devices introduce significant amounts of noise (on the order of 1 to 5 μV RMS).

7.2 *Signal Averaging*

Signal averaging commences after the application of electrodes have been applied to the body surface and the computer starts acquiring the three-lead ECG waveforms. Three principal components to signal averaging include: triggering, averaging itself, and monitoring the noise levels of individual beats and the signal average. In a typical signal averaging system, some patient information, such as name or identifying number, is first entered into the computer. Next, a normal sinus beat QRS complex is selected. This model complex will be used to identify successive normal sinus beats and to synchronize, or time-align, their QRS complexes. After this triggering procedure, the complexes are averaged. By averaging an ensemble of synchronized QRS complexes, the cardiac signal is reinforced and the contaminating noise tends to cancel. During this process, the noise level of each incoming beat is estimated and beats with low enough noise are added to the average. Averaging stops after a fixed number of beats have been processed or after the residual noise in the average reaches a predetermined level.

Figure 7.4–Template selection.

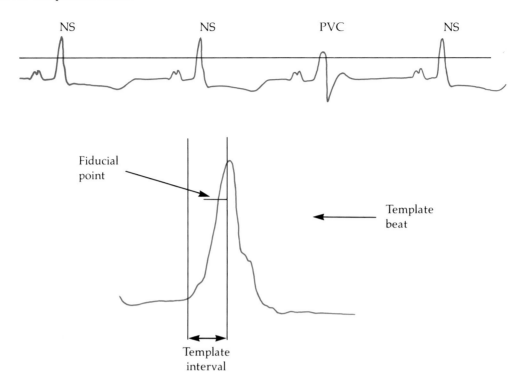

Figure 7.5–Template matching.

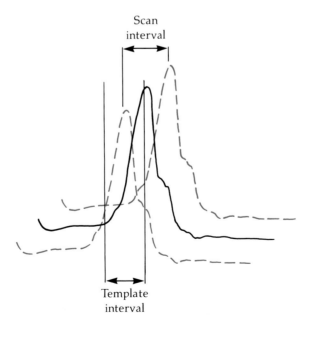

7.2.1   Triggering

The triggering process consists of two steps: template selection and the subsequent matching of each incoming beat to the template. Figure 7.4 illustrates template selection. A rhythm strip with three normal sinus beats (NS) and a premature ventricular contraction (PVC) is shown with an R-wave crossing threshold. Both normal and abnormal QRS complexes are initially detected using a simple hardware device consisting of a bandpass filter (17 to 35 Hz) and a preset level detector. Selection of the template, or model, beat can be performed automatically by the computer or manually by the user. In the latter case, the user selects a beat interactively from a graphical display. This is an effective way of ensuring that a quiet (not noisy) normal sinus beat is chosen. Automatic selection can be problematic when frequent arrhythmias occur. Typically, beats are classified by shape, with the most common occurrence becoming the template.

The function of the template is two-fold. Normal sinus beats must be correctly identified and accurately aligned with the template. The whole QRS complex is needed for accurate identification. Some PVCs may be very similar in some leads to the normal QRS. Fusion beats, for example, differ from normal sinus beats only in the terminal portion of the QRS. The template should be operational in all three of the XYZ leads. For accurate alignment, only a section of the QRS should be used (Figure 7.4). The QR interval is the most distinctive feature of the QRS and usually provides the best alignment model. A period of 40 msec is typical for the template interval. Identifying the fiducial point (Figure 7.4) of later incoming beats remains the objective of template matching.

Figure 7.5 illustrates the basic concept for template matching. The template is drawn with a solid line and the current beat to be aligned with a dotted line. The initial QRS threshold crossing point (Figure 7.4) provides a rough estimate of the fiducial point. The true fiducial point is assumed to lie within a SCAN interval (Figure 7.5). The SCAN interval is usually set to 10 msec, or 5 msec on either side of the initial point detected by the hardware. At each discrete point within the SCAN interval, i.e. every 0.5 or every 1 msec, the *correlation coefficient* is evaluated between the template and the current beat. The time instant of maximum correlation corresponds to the best match between the two. The correlation coefficient, ρ, is given by:

$$\rho = \frac{\sum_{i=1}^{M} x_i y_i}{\sqrt{\sum_{i=1}^{M} x_i^2}\sqrt{\sum_{i=1}^{M} y_i^2}}$$

Equation 7.1

where x_i and y_i represent the template and current beat samples, respectively. The M samples within the 40-msec template interval are used in this computation. Mean removal in the template interval is performed before the cross correlation is computed to optimize the sensitivity of this measure. If the template and the event detected as the current beat are dissimilar in shape, the correlation coefficient has a low value. It ranges from 0 to 1, with a value of 1 signifying a perfect match, i.e., identical waveshapes. A criterion for beat acceptance must be adopted, and is typically a correlation coefficient threshold value of between 0.97 and 0.99. The departure of the correlation coefficient value from 1 relates to timing errors.

Timing errors in the trigger, or fiducial, point do occur. This phenomenon is known as jitter. Four components comprise jitter. First, noise in the ECG causes variance in the correlation coefficient value. Modulation of the ECG waveform by low-frequency respiration artifacts can also shift the fiducial point. Any variability in the QRS waveform morphology tends to lower the correlation coefficient. Lastly, the inter-sample duration (0.5 or 1 msec) places a limit on the accuracy of time alignment. To remove respiration artifacts and to focus on the morphology of the higher frequency QRS components, a highpass filtered version of the QRS can be used for template matching. Attempts to measure trigger jitter are the subject of ongoing reasearch.[148, 149] Correlation measures are insensitive to amplitude. Occasionally PVCs and noise artifacts can exhibit a high degree of correlation with the template. To avoid acceptance of these phenomena, a test is performed on the detected QRS that usually measures its area in the template interval. The area of the current beat must fall within certain bounds, for example, ±10%, of the template area for acceptance.

7.2.2 Signal Averaging Techniques

The technique of signal averaging assumes that a simple mathematical model of the ECG is valid. This model is described by:

$$x(t) = s(t) + n(t)$$

Equation 7.2

where

$x(t)$ is the measured ECG
$s(t)$ is its cardiac signal component
$n(t)$ is the accompanying noise.

The signal and noise components are assumed to be purely additive. The noise alone has a mean value of zero. The signal average of R beats is formed by adding together each beat after triggering, using the fiducial point as an alignment reference. The sum is then divided by R. The signal average, $\bar{x}(t)$, is then described by:

$$\bar{x}(t) = \sum_{i=1}^{R} \frac{x_i(t)}{R}$$

Equation 7.3

where

$\sum$ represents summation
$x_i(t)$ is the ith beat in the ensemble.

This equation becomes:

$$\bar{x}(t) = \sum_{i=1}^{R} \frac{s_i(t) + n_i(t)}{R}$$

Equation 7.4

The signal and noise components appear to be summed independently. Signal averaging assumes that $s_1 = s_i(t) = s(t)$; that is, the signal component of each beat is identical, or purely *deterministic*. The above equation can be simplified to:

$$\bar{x}(t) = s(t) + \sum_{i=1}^{R} \frac{n_i(t)}{R}$$

Equation 7.5

If noise in different beats, for example, $n_1(t)$ and $n_2(t)$, is uncorrelated and has a random distribution, the mean noise value is zero. The noise at any instant is equally likely to be positive or negative. The tendency, therefore, is for the sum of noise values to approach zero. Noise reduction is statistically predictable:[150]

$$\bar{x}(t) = s(t) + \frac{\bar{n}(t)}{\sqrt{R}}$$

Equation 7.6

where $\bar{n}(t)$ is the noise level of a typical beat. Hence, noise is reduced in proportion to the square root of the number of beats averaged. The signal-to-noise ratio (SNR) of a typical individual beat before averaging is described by: $s(t)/\bar{n}(t)$. After averaging, the SNR equals $s(t)/[\bar{n}(t)/\sqrt{R}]$, an improvement of $\sqrt{R}$ times.

Noise reduction remains the sole purpose of signal averaging. The next section considers how the performance of signal averaging can be improved by monitoring noise during the averaging procedure.

7.2.3   Noise Monitoring

The residual noise present in the signal average can be measured after each beat has been added. The following formula provides an *estimate*, $\bar{n}_R(t)$, of the residual noise after R beats have been averaged:

$$\bar{n}_R(t) = \sum_{i=1}^{R} \frac{x_i^2}{R} - \left(\sum_{i=1}^{R} \frac{x_i}{R} \right)^2$$

Equation 7.7

This is only an estimate of the true residual noise because of the latter's random nature. Figure 7.6a presents a graph of the estimated residual noise level during averaging of 300 beats. The noise estimate usually takes about 10 to 30 beats to settle into a predictable form due to the small number of observations available initially.

The averaging process is terminated after a particular residual noise level has been reached. This ensures that different signal averages are of similar quality. Some evidence suggests that a residual noise level of 0.3 µV RMS is sufficient to identify late potentials in almost all recordings.[151,152] The number of beats required to reach this terminal noise level can often be predicted from a noise curve after 10 to 30 beats (Figure 7.6). The residual noise level is proportional to $\sqrt{R}$, the square root of the number of beats averaged. Table 7.1 presents a prediction of the time course of noise reduction. If the projected number of beats required to reach the target noise level is too high, the averaging procedure can be restarted. The usual sources of noise problems include either inadequate electrode application or a restless subject. Table 7.1 shows that the number of beats required to achieve a fixed amount of noise reduction, for example, 0.5 µV, increases rapidly as averaging progresses. In general, in order to halve the residual noise level, four times as many beats must be averaged.

Figure 7.6–Noise monitoring: rejection of adversely noisy beats.

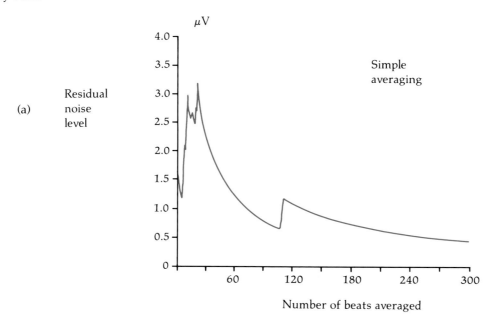

(a)   Residual noise level

μV

Simple averaging

Number of beats averaged

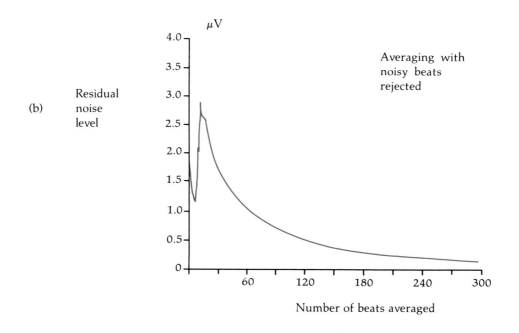

(b)   Residual noise level

μV

Averaging with noisy beats rejected

Number of beats averaged

Table 7.1—Beats required to achieve a fixed amount of noise reduction.

Noise (μV)	Number of Beats
2.0	10
1.0	40
0.5	160
0.3	410

It may not always be possible to reach the target residual noise level. A feasible limit to the averaging duration is about 600 beats, or approximately 7 to 10 minutes. After this, inordinate numbers of beats would be required to achieve further significant reductions in residual noise. Figure 7.6 illustrates a significant problem that can occur with longer averaging times. After about 110 beats, the subject made a sudden arm movement resulting in a very noisy beat being accepted into the average (Figure 7.6a). This beat was not rejected by the template matching procedure. Correlation is robust in the presence of noise. In addition, the template interval may have been quiet. A cough or deep breath correlation might produce a similar noise level. The time course of noise reduction is now significantly retarded.

A method of rejecting such beats, or any adversely noisy beats is highly desirable. Any beat can be rejected if its addition to the signal average does not lower the residual noise. That is:

$$\text{if } \bar{n}_i(t) < \bar{n}_{i-1}(t) \text{ accept ith beat} \qquad \textbf{Equation 7.8}$$

Figure 7.6b shows the effect of implementing this noisy beat rejection scheme.[153] Noise reduction is smooth and continuous. The terminal noise level is always reached with a smaller number of beats, and usually in a shorter time period given a small percentage of rejected beats. This procedure ensures eventual convergence to the target noise level.

7.3 *Time Domain Analysis of the High-Resolution Electrocardiogram*

Figure 7.7 illustrates the steps involved in time domain analysis of the signal-averaged ECG. After averaging, each lead is digitally bandpass filtered and combined to form a vector magnitude waveform. Time and voltage measurements are made on the QRS complex, either from the vector magnitude or individual lead-filtered waveforms. These measurements are first made automatically, but can be manually adjusted. All waveforms, filtered and unfiltered, can be printed on a variety of user-selected scales. Interpretation of the high-resolution ECG is primarily quantitative but it also involves a subjective component. This requires an extension of the electrocardiographer's art: the ability to classify graphic forms. The following sections explore the issues in each step of the high-resolution ECG analysis procedure.

Figure 7.7–Time domain analysis.

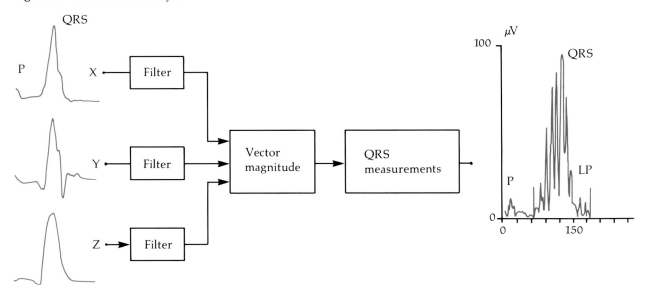

Figure 7.8–Frequency domain characteristics of a filter.

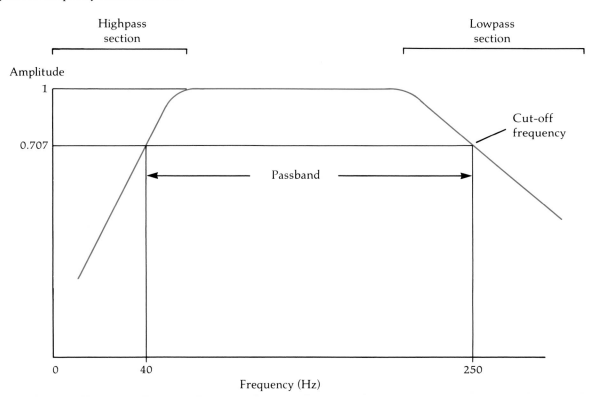

7.3.1   Filtering

Digital filtering of the high-resolution ECG is a complex topic discussed in depth elsewhere.[154] The type of filtering usually applied to the high-resolution ECG is called bandpass. Figure 7.8 illustrates the frequency domain characteristics of a bandpass filter. A bandpass filter consists of two stages: a highpass and a lowpass. The lowpass filter, as its name suggests, passes or does not affect the lower frequencies. The lowpass section (Figure 7.8)has a cut-off frequency of 250 Hz, passing 0.707 of the original signal amplitude at this frequency. Similarly, the highpass section has a cut-off frequency of 40 Hz. The passband is therefore from 40 to 250 Hz. Signal components within this frequency interval are not significantly affected. Signal components outside of this frequency interval are progressively attenuated away from the cut-off frequencies.

From a frequency domain point of view, the ideal filter would have the rectangular shape of the dotted line in Figure 7.8. It would have an infinitely steep roll-off at the cut-off frequencies. Unfortunately, filters introduce distortion into the time domain signal that is directly proportional to the steepness of the roll-off. The design objective for high-resolution ECG filters is to minimize this distortion while attaining adequate frequency discrimination to isolate late potentials. For practical purposes, this problem is restricted to the highpass section where much greater frequency discrimination (that is, a steeper roll-off) is needed to separate late potentials from the ST segment. The ECG is considered as a time signal, with waves and intervals whose shapes and durations, respectively, aid in the interpretation of the ECG. A filter is judged by its performance in separating these waves and allowing accurate measurements, with its frequency domain characteristics of secondary importance.

Different design methods exist for digital filters currently in use with the high-resolution ECG. Figure 7.9 shows the application of two different filter types to the same data. Figure 7.9a results from applying a fourth order Butterworth filter in a bi-directional mode.[155] The filter is applied in forward time from the start of the record to the mid-point of the QRS. It is then applied in reverse time from the end of the record to the mid-point of the QRS. This type of filter causes a distortion know as "ringing" in the direction of the filter only. Therefore, the QRS complex is distorted, but the onset and offset points are well preserved. In some cases, ringing of the P wave may obscure the QRS onset. Figure 7.9b shows the application of a spectral window filter. This filter causes much less distortion (note the preserved PR interval) but spreads the QRS complex. The amount of spreading depends on the filter design. For the filter shown, the difference in QRS offset between the two filters is 3 msecs.

A breakdown of the advantages and disadvantages of these filters is given elsewhere.[154] Essentially, the shape of filtered waves is heavily distorted by the bi-directional filter, leading to inaccurate amplitude measurements. It may optimally define the QRS offset, if this point is not corrupted by ringing of the ST segment noise. The spectral window filter always smears the major waves, leading to some errors in QRS offset. This error can range from 0 to 15 msecs for a typical 40 Hz filter. The exact value depends on the filter design. A good filter can restrict the error in almost all cases to less than 5 msecs.[154] Smearing increases when the QRS ends abruptly. Unlike the bi-directional filter, the filtered waveshape is an accurate rendering of the waveshape in the passband of the filter.

The frequency spectrum of late potentials is unknown in any individual patient. Applying filters with different frequency responses leads to different results. Figure 7.10d il-

Figure 7.9–Differences in digital filter types.

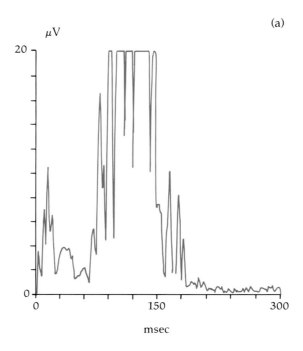

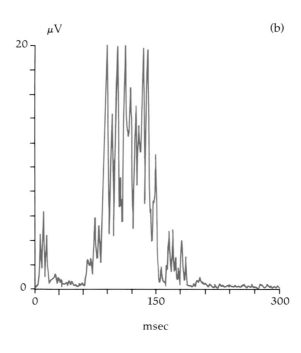

Figure 7.10–Applying filters with different cut-off frequencies.

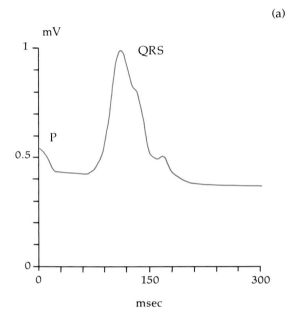

(a)

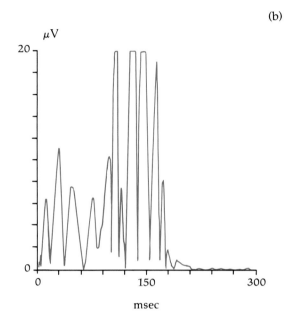

(b)

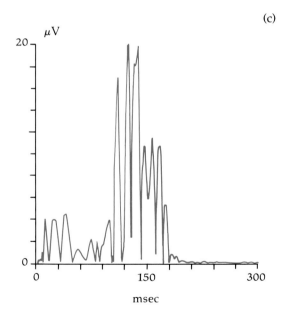

(c)

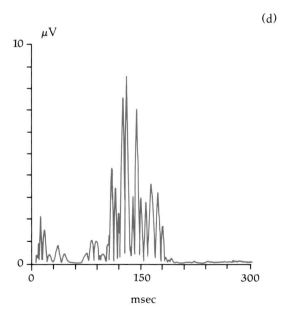

(d)

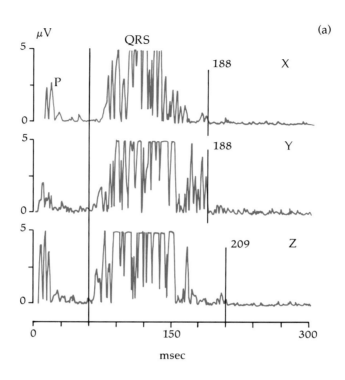

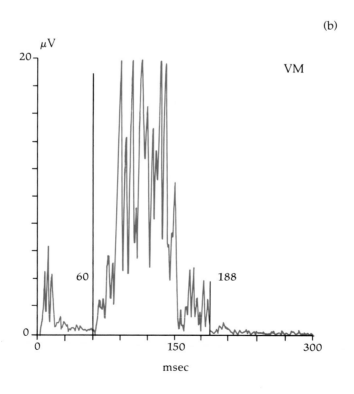

lustrates the use of bandpass filters with highpass cut-off frequencies of (b) 25, (c) 40, and (d) 80 Hz. Figure 7.10a has not been digitally filtered; its passband is 0.05 to 300 Hz. A late potential at the very end of the QRS, evident in Figure 7.10b, is reduced in amplitude as the filter cut-off frequency rises. A progressive underestimation of the QRS offset occurs in Figure 7.10 b through d. (note that Figure 7.10d is scaled twice as much as Figure 7.10 b and c). These data were obtained with the bi-directional filter described above.

Ringing of the P wave obscures the QRS onset at lower highpass cut-off frequencies (25 and 40 Hz). These filters have a heavier action in that their highpass roll-offs are steeper (Figure 7.9). A light filter, such as a simple difference filter, generally pinpoints the QRS onset accurately.[154]

7.3.2 Vector Magnitude Transform

Recording three orthogonal XYZ leads allows their combination into a single vector magnitude waveform VM(t). This transformation is illustrated in Figure 7.11. After digital filtering, the three resultant XYZ leads are combined using:

$$VM(t) = \sqrt{X^2(t) + Y^2(t) + Z^2(t)}$$

Equation 7.9

This transformation simplifies analysis by reducing the information to one waveform. However, the vector magnitude has a degraded signal-to-noise ratio, compared to the individual XYZ leads.[156] This leads to an underestimation of the QRS offset, as illustrated in Figure 7.11. The QRS duration measured in the longest individual lead (Z) is 149 msec, as opposed to 128 msec in the vector magnitude.

7.3.3 Automatic Measurements

Figure 7.12 shows the automatic measurements that are commonly made from the vector magnitude waveform. These include the QRS onset, offset and duration, the amplitude of the terminal 40 msecs (RMS40) and the duration of the low amplitude signal (LAS) below 40 µV.

The QRS onset is easily detected from the absolute spatial velocity vector. A large increase in signal level is present at the end of the PQ interval. This simple filter removes the low-level trend of the PR interval and causes no P wave spreading. The high resolution QRS onset occurs 10-20ms earlier than that detected in the conventional ECG. This is due to the inclusion of conducting system activity, notably from the left bundle branch and Purkinje fibres, which generate a signal of up to 20 µv in amplitude.[157]

The QRS offset is determined relative to the noise level of the filtered ST segment. An estimate of the noise level is made in a "reference window", typically of about 40 msecs duration, as illustrated in Figure 7.12. The ST segment is then searched retrospectively until the measured noise level in a moving "search window" (Figure 7.12) exceeds the reference window noise by some factor, typically a three-fold increase. The QRS offset is hence defined statistically, similarly to a chi-squared test. The design objective of QRS offset detection algorithms is to maximize the number of degrees of freedom. Simply translated, the search procedure should be sensitive to low-level signals and as specific (noise insensitive) as possible. Detection sensitivity and specificity are directly traded off against each other. A shorter search window increases detection sensitivity but is susceptible to

Figure 7.12–QRS measurements.

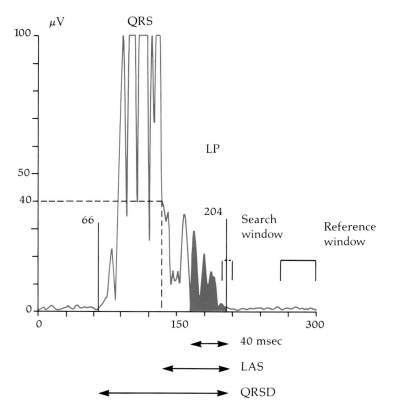

Figure 7.13–Time periods for spectral analysis.

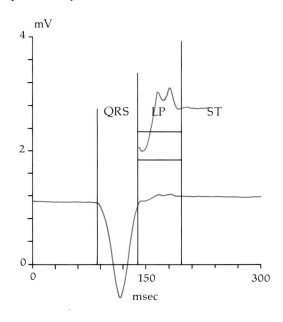

noise spikes. A similar effect is achieved by use of the median value in the search window, and by lowering the noise threshold factor. A cosinusoidal window gives better performance than a rectangular window if the noise is homogeneous. More sophisticated noise detection algorithms have been reported, based on the techniques above.[158]

The QRS duration is found simply from the QRS offset and onset values. The RMS40 value is calculated in the shaded area of Figure 7.12; unlike the QRS duration it depends heavily on the chosen QRS offset. A change in offset of a few msecs typically causes a less than 5% change in QRS duration, but up to a 50% change in RMS40 value. The LAS duration is indicated in Figure 7.12. It exhibits a susceptibility to noise similar to RMS40.

7.4 *Interpretation of Late Potentials*

Qualitatively, a late potential is characterized as a low-level tail that is either a part of, or separate from, the terminal QRS. Most researchers have developed criteria for late potentials using a particular filter and critical values of QRS duration, RMS40, and LAS. Highpass filter cut-off frequencies of 25, 40, and 80 Hz have been used with a majority of researchers choosing the 40 Hz filter. Critical values of QRS duration greater than 120 msecs or 114 msecs, RMS40 less than 25 µV or 20 µV, and LAS (below 40 µV) greater than 38 msecs have been used to define the presence of late potentials. These measurements have been examined together in various combinations. They have also been used in conjunction with measures of ventricular performance and ventricular ectopy. The clinical performances of the different approaches described above have been reviewed.[145]

Both commercial and research signal averaging systems implement noise measurement, filtering, and QRS offset detection in different ways. The computer programs that perform these tasks are for the most part unpublished. It is difficult to compare these procedures in different machines directly. For example, protocol for averaging to 0.3 µV residual noise and application of a 40 to 250 Hz bandpass filter can result in significantly different results with different signal averaging systems. Measurement algorithms for QRS onset and offset are prone to error. Manual adjustment is frequently required by the user. A high-resolution graphical display is needed for this operation. It is also important QRS onset is selected from a display of the absolute spatial velocity vector to avoid problems of P wave ringing (bi-directional filter) or smearing (spectral window filter).

7.5 *Frequency Domain Analysis of the High-Resolution Electrocardiogram*

The idea of frequency domain or spectral analysis of the high-resolution ECG has been explored by many authors. The rationale for this approach is that it may obviate the need for filtering. The interpretation of late potentials via the frequency spectrum was first proposed by Cain.[159] Frequency domain analysis of the high-resolution ECG is a complex topic that has been explored in some depth.[160] This presentation is an intuitive approach to understanding the techniques and limitations of spectral analysis of the high-resolution ECG.

Figure 7.14–Power spectra of different ECG time periods.

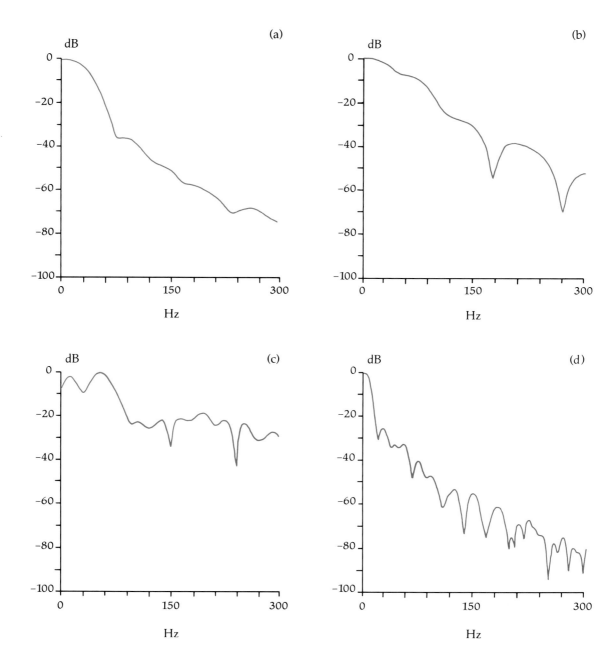

Figure 7.15–Effects of windows.

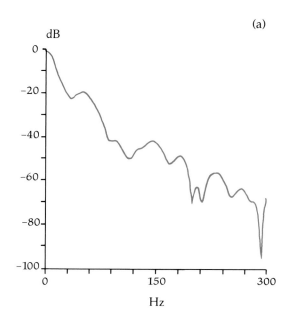

(a)

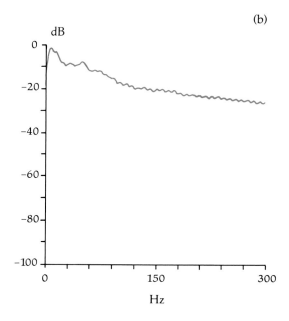

(b)

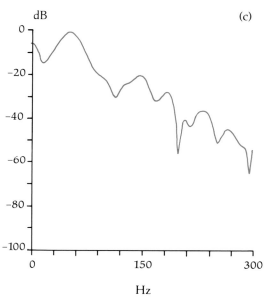

(c)

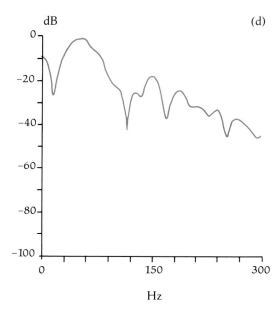

(d)

Figure 7.16–Spectrotemporal mapping.

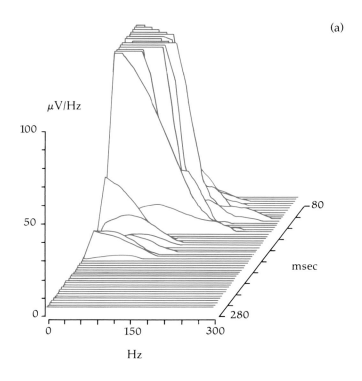

(a)

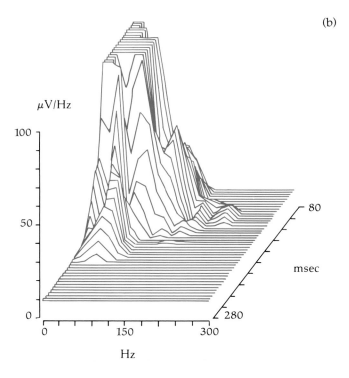

(b)

7.5.1 Techniques

With one or two exceptions[161], spectral analysis of the high-resolution ECG has been performed using classical techniques. It is essentially a four-step procedure: a time period is selected for analysis; the data in this interval is possibly filtered in some manner, usually by removal of the DC value; the data is then multiplied by a window function; and the power spectrum is computed, typically with a computer algorithm known as the Fast-Fourier transform.

Figure 7.13 illustrates a logical choice of possible ECG intervals to analyze: the QRS, late potential (LP), and ST segment periods. In practice, the optimal period to analyze is unknown. Figure 7.14 illustrates the spectra resulting from analysis of the QRS, the late potentials, the ST segment, and the entire period encompassing these three features. The spectra are plotted on a decibel scale. Compared to 0 dB, the value at -20 dB is down by a factor of 10, at -40 dB it is down by a factor of 100, and so forth. The data is only meaningful above -60 or -70 dB. Several observations can be made from these traces. First, the spectrum of the late potentials is nondescript. It is smoother than the other spectra because its *spectral resolution* is lower. The spectrum of the ST segment in reality does not extend beyond about 30 Hz. The apparent power in the spectrum above this frequency is due to windowing artifacts. The spectrum of the QRS + LP + ST period is a weighted sum of the previous three individual spectra. The contribution of each of these spectra is weighted in direct proportion to both the amplitude and duration of the time signals. Since late potentials are short-lived low-level signals, their contribution is minimal (less than 0.1%). The spectrum of Figure 7.14d is predominantly influenced by the QRS. In summary, the exact choice of time interval to analyze has a major impact on the spectral representation of late potentials.

Figure 7.15 illustrates the effect on the spectrum of other technical aspects. Figures 7.15a and 7.15b show the spectrum of a 120-msec interval, beginning at the LP waveform and extending into the ST segment, due to the Blackman-Harris and rectangular window functions, respectively. The choice of window radically affects the shape of the spectrum. Figure 7.15c shows the spectrum of the filtered data (40 to 250 Hz). The predominant influence of the ST segment is removed. However, the spectral peak at about 60 Hz, which is present in all four traces, is a windowing artifact. Figure 7.15d demonstrates the spectrum of the filtered data after placing the window 10 msecs to the right. The lower frequency portion of the spectrum (0 to 60 Hz) changes significantly, reflecting the instability of the power spectrum.

7.5.2 Spectrotemporal Mapping

The frequency spectrum of the high-resolution ECG varies continuously with time. The power variation of the high-resolution ECG in both time and frequency can be seen by spectrotemporal mapping (STM).[160] This is performed by sliding a fixed-length window across the ECG waveform in small time increments and computing a sequence of spectra.

Figure 7.16 illustrates two STMs with window lengths of 16 msecs and 64 msecs. Data are displayed on a magnitude scale. Data values below 1 μV/Hz are clipped, or set equal to zero, to emphasize the contours of the display. The STMs are computed over a 280-msec interval consisting of the QRS and LP components and most of the ST segment. Frequency ranges from 0 to 300 Hz. In Figure 7.16a the 16-msec window localizes power in time but affords little spectral resolution. In Figure 7.16b a greater spectral resolution results but adjacent spectra are less distinct on the time axis. Both STMs attempt to represent the *time-frequency structure* of the high-resolution ECG. Their ability to do this is limited because resolution in one domain, that is, time or frequency, is inversely proportional to resolution in the other domain. The desired time-frequency resolution is on the order of 10 msecs and 10 Hz. The resolution in these intervals is limited to approximately one-tenth of this desired resolution,[160] due to the nature of time-frequency representations. The time resolution (T) and frequency resolution (B) are related by:

$$TB \approx 3.6$$
Equation 7.10

For a time interval of 120 msecs, the minimum resolvable bandwidth is about 30 Hz. If the period of each STM time window increases, the bandwidth over which a significant power value can be resolved decreases. Conversely, if the time interval is decreased, say to 60 msecs, the resolvable bandwidth increases to 60 Hz. This relationship is known as the uncertainty principle. If the time-frequency structure of the high-resolution ECG is too fine for the uncertainty principle (that is, if its spectrum is varying too rapidly with time), then no spectral analysis technique can decompose the waveform.

The spectrum of the high-resolution ECG is unstable because it is continuously varying with time. Therefore, the position of the window is very important and significantly affects the computed spectrum. Late potentials contribute much less to the spectrum than the ST segment or normal QRS waveforms because of their low amplitude and short duration. Some form of filtering before spectral analysis, therefore, seems advisable to reduce the influence of the ST segment, in particular. However, the initial motive for using spectral analysis was precisely to avoid this.

The principal obstacle to spectral analysis techniques is the limited spectral resolution available with the high-resolution ECG. This concept becomes clearer when the spectral analysis technique is considered as another means of filtering.[162] Although considerable interest in spectral analysis of the high-resolution ECG exists, the issues and limitations discussed above suggest that time domain techniques should provide a better analysis of late potentials.

8.0   ELECTROPHYSIOLOGY

The remarkable progress achieved in the past two decades in the diagnosis and treatment of complex cardiac rhythm disturbances has occurred through advances in the field of cardiac electrophysiology. In this section, cardiac electrophysiologic studies are outlined. These studies include surface and intracavitary electrograms to record the electrical activity of the heart, programmed electrical stimulation to assess conduction tissue properties and to induce atrial or ventricular arrhythmias, and cardiac mapping to localize the site of the abnormal rhythm. The transesophageal method for pacing the heart and recording the left atrial electrogram offers another technique that can hold diagnostic and therapeutic significance.

Surgical and nonsurgical interventions for correcting rhythmic disturbances are described. Radiofrequency catheter ablation, a nonsurgical method, is becoming the procedure of choice for Wolff-Parkinson-White syndromes and atrioventricular node ablation or modification. Applications for use of direct current shock, such as cardioversion and defibrillation, are also presented. The implantable cardioverter-defibrillator, designed to treat ventricular tachycardia and ventricular fibrillation, is being refined both in application and design. In the future, cardiologists may have the capability to implant these cardioverter-defibrillator devices in a catheterization laboratory setting.

8.1 *Electrophysiology Equipment Requirements*

Four types of equipment used for performing electrophysiologic studies are illustrated in Figure 8.1. Single-plane fluoroscopy is used in most electrophysiology studies. The increasing complexity of interventional electrophysiology procedures is demonstrated by multiplane fluoroscopy with 7- and 9-inch magnification. It is advisable to use cineangiography and digital processing for interventional cases, however.

8.1.1 Recording Devices

Catheters provide direct contact with the endocardial surface of the heart. Introduced through a major vein or artery of the body, catheters record electrograms and stimulate the heart through their multiple electrodes. The catheters are usually made of woven Dacron of 5-, 6-, or 7-F diameter. Multiple (2 to 10) platinum-ring electrodes with variable interelectrode spacing (2-, 5-, 10-millimeters) are located at the distal portion of the catheter. The most frequently used catheters are 6-F quadripolar catheters with 5- to 10-millimeters interelectrode spacing (Figure 8.2). Deflectable-tip catheters, more recent introductions, are very useful for mapping and ablation techniques.

The multiple pins at the proximal ends of the catheters are connected to a switch box, which directs the incoming electrogram signals to the amplifier. Through the switch box, stimulator pulses can be directed to the desired bipole at any given location.

Amplifiers receive and process the electrogram signals obtained through the catheter. They have frequency filters, amplitude gain, signal limiters, and calibration markers. Filtering of the intracardiac signals depends on the catheter location. Filtering capability should be in the range of 10 to 1000 Hz. The desirable amplification ranges between 0.5 and 20 mV, and the amplifiers should have minimal noise at sensitivities of 0.02 to 0.05 mV/cm.

The electrical signals from the amplifier are displayed on a multichannel oscilloscope or monitor. This monitor should be easily visible to the operator and should also have storage (freeze-frame) and triggering capabilities. Recordings can print directly onto paper through a multichannel strip chart recorder, stored in FM magnetic tape recorders, or digitized and saved on optical disks. The multichannel paper strip chart recorder should have variable recording speeds, ranging from 10 mm/sec to 200 mm/sec. Computerized systems that have recently become available can digitize the incoming signal and allow its processing, manipulation, and storage.

8.1.2 Stimulator for Cardiac Pacing

The cardiac stimulator should have the following capabilities: Deliver constant current impulses of variable duration (commonly 2-msec duration) at variable current intensities (0 to 20 mA) (the recommended current intensity used in intracardiac stimulation is twice the myocardial diastolic threshold); sense the intracardiac electrogram signal for synchro-

Figure 8.1–Schematic drawing of an electrophysiology laboratory.

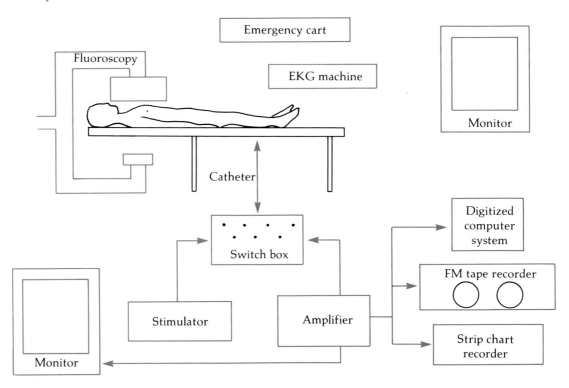

Figure 8.2–Examples of electrode catheters.

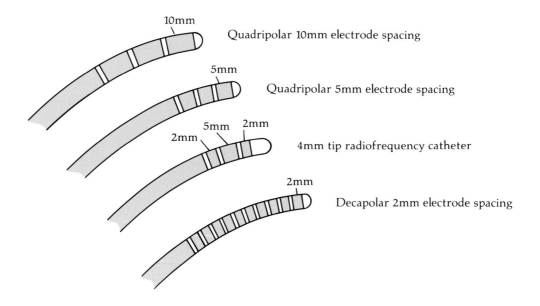

nization; have continuous and interrupted pacing capabilities; and deliver up to three extra stimuli, at adjustable coupling intervals, to the sensed or paced rhythm.

8.2   *Surface Electrograms*

The electrical conduction properties of tissues surrounding the heart make it possible for electrical activity generated by the heart to be recorded at the body surface. This forms the basis of electrocardiography.

In routine electrophysiology studies, three to six surface electrograms are used in conjunction with intracardiac signals. Selecting surface leads allows the frontal and horizontal electrical plane axes of a given rhythm to be determined. Common lead combinations are I, AVF and V_1, or I, III and V_1. The capability to rapidly change the displayed leads has advantage. One should also have 12-lead electrocardiographic recording capabilities, particularly for pace mapping.

8.3   *Intracavitary Electrograms*

The catheters placed in direct contact with the endocardial surface of the heart detect the electrical events that occur between their electrodes. During a routine electrophysiology study, the catheters are positioned inside the heart in the following manner (Figure 8.3): One catheter is placed in the high right atrium near the junction with the superior vena cava. This catheter records the electrical activity of the atrium immediately after activity is generated by the sinus node. A second catheter is positioned across the tricuspid valve. Part of the catheter overrides the tricuspid annulus near the membranous ventricular septum and records signals of both the lower right atrium and the right ventricle. Because it is adjacent to the atrioventricular (AV) node and bundle of His, a "His electrogram" is recorded with the catheter in this position. Conduction times through the AV node and Purkinje system result from measuring the AH and HV intervals (Figure 8.4). For adequate recording at the bundle of His, the amplifiers must be set with filtering between 25 and 250 Hz. A third catheter is located in the apex of the right ventricle. For ventricular stimulation protocols, this catheter can move to the right ventricular outflow tract position.

For electrophysiologic studies in patients with supraventricular arrhythmias, a multipolar catheter is usually positioned in the coronary sinus. The coronary sinus ostium lies in the low posterior right atrium. The coronary sinus is situated behind the left AV mitral ring, allowing the recording of both left atrial and left ventricular events. Special mapping techniques allow the recording of accessory pathway potentials. For electrophysiologic mapping, regular or deflectable-tip catheters can be manipulated by fluoroscopy to any desired position in the heart. Local electrograms should be recorded.

8.4   *Programmed Stimulation*

Programmed electrical stimulation was introduced in 1971 by Wellens and now operates as an integral and essential component of clinical electrophysiology studies. Programmed electrical stimulation assesses the conduction tissue properties (for example, refractory periods) for induction of atrial or ventricular arrhythmias. It consists of a six to eight-beat train (S1) of atrial or ventricular pacing (drive) at a predetermined rate (100 to 150 bpm)

Figure 8.3–Catheter positioning for intracavitary electrograms.

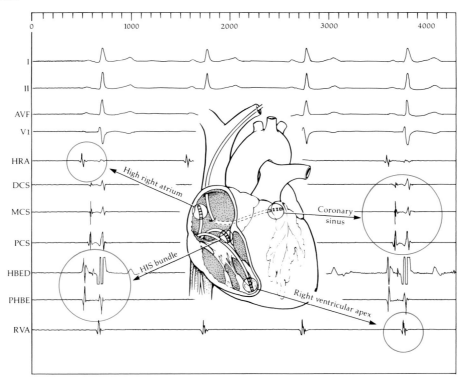

Figure 8.4–Recording of AH-HV interval.

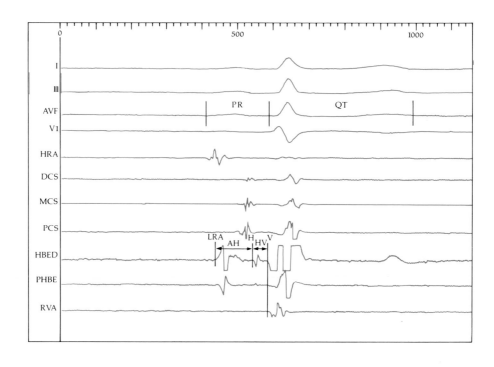

followed by a premature extra-stimulus (S2) (Figure 8.5a). The coupling interval (S1-S2) between the last drive beat (S1) and the premature depolarization (S2) is progressively shortened by 10 to 20 msec until it fails to capture in the paced tissue.

Two (-S2S3) or three (-S2S3S4) extra stimuli can be used to induce arrhythmias (Figures 8.5b and 8.5c). By sequentially shortening the coupling interval between S3-S4, S2-S3, and S1-S2, the entire diastolic period is scanned for vulnerability. If one uses more than three extra-stimuli, nonspecific responses of little clinical value are obtained. Programmed electrical stimulation is a systematic process and should be applied at least at two different sites in the right ventricle at two drive-cycle lengths (or rates) to satisfy the minimum criteria for induction of ventricular tachycardia. The induced ventricular tachycardia must be identical to that spontaneously documented previously. Occasionally, this technique can unmask other previously elusive arrhythmias.

8.5 *Cardiac Mapping*

Through cardiac mapping, the zone in the heart responsible for the initiation and perpetuation of an abnormal rhythm is localized. With this technique, the heart is "mapped" by an exhaustive and complete recording of electrograms. Cardiac mapping usually is first performed in the cardiac catheterization laboratory, then later in the operating room when the heart can be exposed. In the electrophysiology laboratory, cardiac mapping is achieved by obtaining samples of electrograms from sites in the heart chamber where an abnormal circuit is known to originate and travel. Bipolar and, occasionally, unipolar electrograms are recorded from the mapping catheter. This catheter is manipulated to different sites under fluoroscopic guidance.

Usually, cardiac mapping is performed during induced tachycardia. The earliest "site of activation" is the position of interest (Figure 8.6). Mapping can also be done during sinus rhythm, either to localize areas of slow conduction or to record accessory pathway potentials.

In cases of ventricular tachycardia, the cardiac chambers most commonly mapped are the left and right ventricles. In cases of Wolff-Parkinson-White syndrome, the coronary sinus and the right AV ring are mapped. Right or left atrial mapping is occasionally used in ectopic atrial rhythms.

During cardiac surgery, the heart is exposed and direct positioning of epicardial or endocardial electrodes can take place. Surgery for arrhythmias depends on accurate localization of the arrhythmogenic area or the aberrant conduction tissue in the heart. Initially, surgeons utilized a manually mobilized electrode probe for direct mapping. This was a laborious and time consuming process, however, prolonging surgery and increasing the risk of complications. During the past few years, computerized multiplexing mapping systems have been developed. These computerized systems allow simultaneous electrogram recordings of 64, 128, or 256 areas, depending on the software used. A computerized reconstruction of activation maps allows for rapid determination of the earliest electrogram activity, which easily correlates to an anatomical site.

Devices such as socks, balloons, and bands with imbedded electrodes have produced faster mapping of epicardial, endocardial, or AV groove areas of the heart, respectively. Computerized multiplexing mapping systems have simplified and shortened surgical procedures and helped to improve the surgical success rate.

Figure 8.5–Ventricular programmed stimulation.

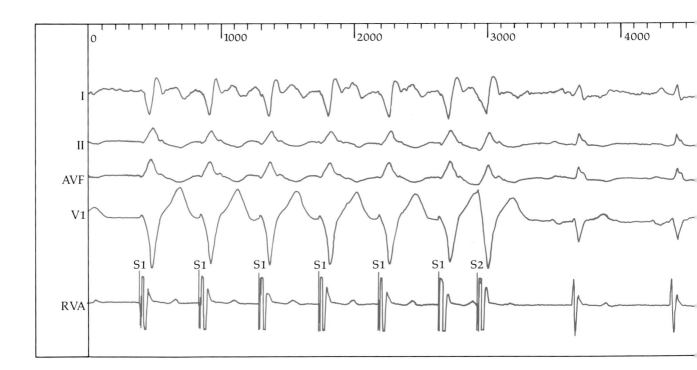

Figure 8.6–Example of ventricular mapping during orthodromic reciprocating tachycardia for Wolff-Parkinson-White syndrome.

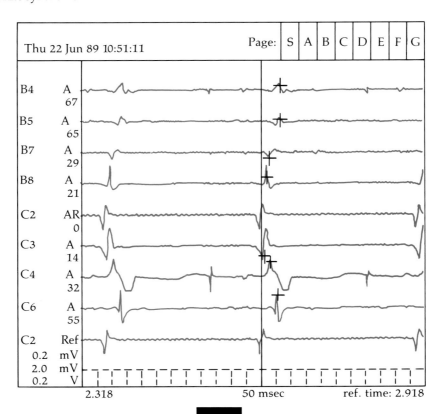

8.6 *Radiofrequency Catheter Ablation*

Percutaneous catheter ablation techniques, introduced in 1982, have made it possible to interrupt an AV or accessory pathway conduction or to destroy a ventricular tachycardia focus without the need for surgical intervention. In the initial catheter ablation procedures, high-energy direct current shocks were delivered through a catheter. Although the success rate with these procedures was acceptable, they had the disadvantage of requiring general anesthesia. These procedures allowed little control over the amount of damage caused by barotrauma. To overcome such disadvantages, lower energy shock and radiofrequency techniques have been developed, and have achieved good success rates.

The radiofrequency impulses used in cardiac electrophysiology are continuous, unmodulated sine waves at 550 Hz with variable outputs (between 0 and 50 V). The impulses are applied through a catheter with a 4-mm platinum tip. The radiofrequency energy delivered through the catheter is converted into heat. Because the point of maximal generated heat occupies the interface between the tissue and the catheter tip, good tissue contact is mandatory for successful results. Tissue injury depends on the amount of current density and the time of exposure. During radiofrequency procedures, the average voltage is between 30 and 50 V, the current between 0.30 and 0.60 A, and the power lies between 10 and 30 W. The exposure time is 10 to 40 seconds. Monitoring of catheter temperature and/or impedance provides information regarding tissue contact and coagulation around the electrode.

Special deflectable catheters with 4-mm tip electrodes are used for radiofrequency ablation. These catheters aid in positioning the catheter at the precise ablation site in the heart. Radiofrequency ablation is rapidly becoming the procedure of choice in the treatment of Wolff-Parkinson-White syndromes and AV node ablation. Its application in cases of ventricular tachycardia remains still under investigation.

8.7 *Transesophageal Pacing and Recording*

The concept of transesophageal recording and pacing results from the close anatomical relationship that exists between the esophagus and the left atrium. Recording of the left atrial electrogram and pacing of the heart offers both diagnostic and therapeutic information.

Transesophageal recording and pacing is accomplished by positioning bipolar electrodes in the esophagus at the level of the left atrium. The electrode catheter can be advanced either through a nasogastric tube or directly through the nostrils. Usually, an "esophageal pill" attached to a fine cable is swallowed by an awake and cooperative patient. The capsule dissolves, and the bipolar electrode rests at the desired location in the esophagus. The electrogram, preamplified with a high-pass filter to improve signal quality, is recorded through a standard electrocardiography machine (Figure 8.7). This minimally invasive technique has many benefits in clinical practice. Recording of atrial activity permits timing of atrial and ventricular events. Thus, ventricular and supraventricular arrhythmias can be quickly and inexpensively differentiated. Based on the information obtained, therapy for the specific arrhythmia can proceed.

Transesophageal pacing of the left atrium requires both a higher pulse width (10 msec) and current intensity (20 to 40 mA) than intracavitary pacing because of the distance between the esophagus and the left atrium. This type of pacing can overdrive and

Figure 8.7–Esophageal electrocardiography.

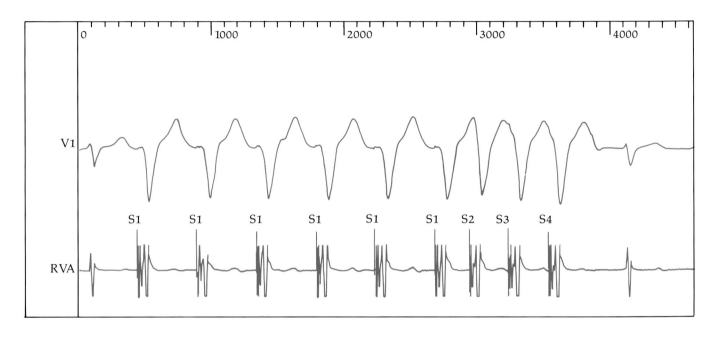

Figure 8.8–Location of synchronization for cardioversion.

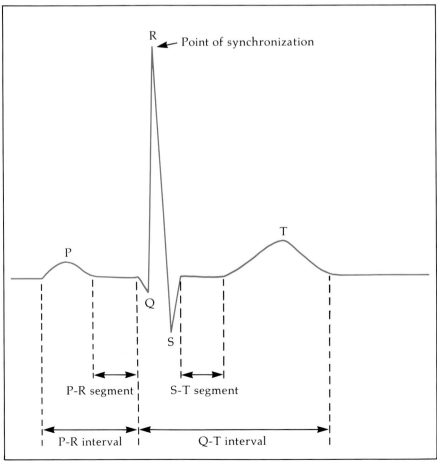

terminate supraventricular arrhythmias of re-entry mechanisms. Because of the distance factor, this pacing technique is more effective in children than in adults.

8.8 *Cardioversion*

Cardioversion, a method for interrupting cardiac rhythm disturbances, utilizes direct current shock synchronized to the QRS complex. The point of synchronization is located in the peak of the R wave (Figure 8.8). Synchronization avoids delivering the electric shock during the T wave, which represents myocardial repolarization. Electrical inhomogeneity can occur, sometimes causing the induction of more serious arrhythmias if a nonsynchronized shock is delivered in this vulnerable period. The electric shock delivered during the QRS complex depolarizes all excitable myocardium and restores electrical homogeneity, thus terminating the arrhythmias and allowing the appearance of normal rhythm and conduction. Variable amounts of energy are required, depending on the type of rhythm to be converted. Equipment should have the capability of delivering up to 360 joules of direct current energy.

Patients undergoing cardioversion usually receive either a short-acting sedative or a short-term, light anesthesia administered intravenously. An attempt is made to produce enough amnesia so that the patient will not remember the actual electrical shock. The energy dosage varies according to the type of arrhythmia treated. For example, atrial flutter requires less energy than does atrial fibrillation and ventricular tachycardia requires less energy than does ventricular fibrillation. Elective cardioversion is performed with monitoring equipment and an emergency cart readily available. Patients usually undergo cardioversion on an outpatient basis.

8.9 *Defibrillation*

Defibrillation, or the application of direct current shock without synchronization, is used during a cardiac emergency. Defibrillation converts rhythms that are too fast or too disorganized to be synchronized by currently available equipment (Figure 8.9). Such rhythms include ventricular flutter or ventricular fibrillation. In ventricular fibrillation, defibrillation is more effective if the metabolic state, including acidosis, is corrected.

Defibrillation is carried out at the scene of cardiac arrest (for example, in a patient's home), during emergency transfer, or in the hospital setting. The patient is usually unconscious and in a state of serious hemodynamic compromise.

The success of defibrillation results from the sudden depolarization of a critical myocardial mass and the capability of the current to stop the fibrillation wavefront. Proper positioning of the defibrillator paddles is important. Direct current with biphasic waveforms is more efficacious than monophasic waveforms of the same duration. Defibrillation usually requires higher energy shocks than does cardioversion because of the nature of the arrhythmia.

8.10 *Implantable Cardioverter-Defibrillator*

For two decades, Mirowski and colleagues at The Johns Hopkins University applied the experience and knowledge obtained from external defibrillation to the development and refinement of an implantable cardioverter-defibrillator (ICD). The device was approved

Figure 8.9–Polymorphic ventricular tachycardia.
An example of disorganized rhythm.

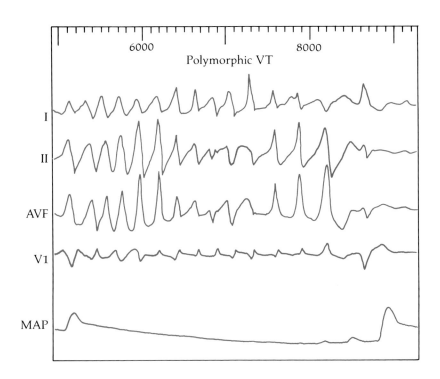

for clinical use in 1986. Since then, more than 20,000 ICDs have been implanted in patients worldwide. Components of the currently available ICD are shown in Figure 8.10.

To be eligible to receive an ICD, a patient must have had at least one episode of ventricular fibrillation or hemodynamically compromising ventricular tachycardia. Extensive electrophysiologic studies are performed before implantation to determine whether the ventricular arrhythmias can be reproducibly induced, to assess their cycle length, and to define the degree of hemodynamic compromise. Adequate programming of the ICD results in this information.

The implantation procedure is performed by a cardiac surgeon with the patient under general anesthesia. Although various surgical approaches can expose the surface of the heart, a left lateral thoracotomy is commonly used. Once the surface of the heart is exposed, the two rate-sensing leads are placed a short distance from each other and fixed to the epicardial surface of the right or left ventricle. To achieve reliable rate sensing, these leads must sense an R wave amplitude equal to or greater than 5 mV. Pacing threshold and R wave signal duration are recommended for positioning the leads. After the leads are in place, two defibrillator patches are located over the heart or pericardium, usually anteriorly and posteriorly. The patches should encompass the largest possible amount of healthy heart muscle. Ventricular tachycardia or fibrillation is then induced by programmed electrical stimulation or alternating current stimulation. The defibrillation threshold (the minimum energy required to correct the induced arrhythmia) is determined by delivering a specific amount of direct current through an external cardioverter-defibrillator. In most centers, the acceptable threshold for reproducible defibrillation is 15 joules or less. Once satisfactory rate sensing and an acceptable defibrillation threshold occur, the cables from these leads are tunneled to the front of the abdomen. An opening or pocket large enough to accommodate the generator is created in the space between the fat and the abdominal muscles. The device is then connected to the patches and rate-sensing leads. Ventricular fibrillation is again induced for final testing of the ICD before completion of the procedure.

Currently, the following types of ICDs are under development:

- Devices with various programmable energy discharges designed to treat ventricular tachycardia at a lower energy than that required for ventricular fibrillation.

- Devices with antitachycardia pacing algorithms and bradycardia backup pacing through which overdrive pacing can be used to treat the arrhythmia before direct current shocks are delivered.

- Devices that could be implanted in the catheterization laboratory by the cardiologist. Clinical studies are under way to test these.

The commercially available ICD is still quite large. It weighs about 240 grams and resembles a deck of cards in size. Currently, available data reveal that the ICD has been successful in preventing sudden cardiac death in many cases. The actual shock is usually delivered when the patient is unconscious, except in cases of hemodynamically-tolerated ventricular tachycardia in which small amounts of energy are used for cardioversion of this arrhythmia in a conscious patient.

Figure 8.10–Schematic drawing of the implantable cardioverter-defibrillator (ICD). (a) Battery unit containing two capacitors capable of providing a maximum energy discharge of 31 J. (b) Two defibrillation patches placed on opposing surfaces of the heart. (c) Two rate-sensing leads that monitor the heart rate and determine the need for defibrillation.

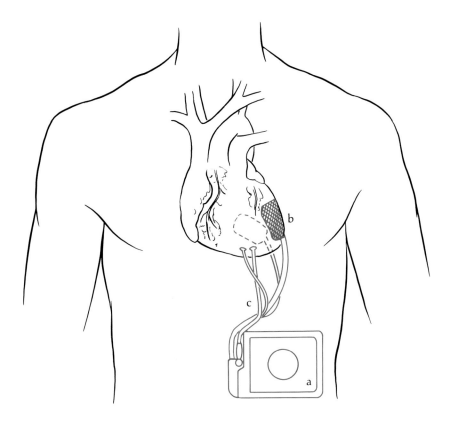

9.0   ABBREVIATIONS

AAMI Association for the Advancement of Medical Instrumentation

AC alternating current

A/D alternating/direct current ratio

AHA American Heart Association

AICD automatic implantable cardioverter-defibrillator

AMI acute myocardial infarction

AMP ampere

AVESTD Magid Statistic (or SDIndex)

AV atrioventricular

AZTEC Amplitude-Zone-Time-Epoch-Coding

B frequency resolution

bpm beats per minute

CANS central autonomic nervous system

CCAVB congenital complete AV block

CHF congestive heart failure

cm centimeter

COMP computer

DC direct current

DFT Discrete-Fourier transform

DFT/FFT Fast-Fourier transform of the DFT procedure

DSP digital signal processor

Ebp esophageal lead

ECG electrocardiogram

ECRI Emergency Care Research Institute

EKG electrocardiogram

Electrodes (in vectorcardiography)

   A positive electrode located at left midaxillary line

   C positive electrode located midway between the left midaxillary line and over the sternum

   CC5 negative electrode on the right of the chest

   CH5 negative electrode on the head

   CM2 negative electrode to the left sternal border at the junction of the fifth rib

   CM5 negative electrode on the manubrium

   CR5 negative electrode on the right arm

   CS5 negative electrode on the right shoulder

   E positive electrode over the sternum

   H positive electrode on the head

   I positive electrode on the right midaxillary line

   M positive electrode on the spine

EP pediatric electrophysiologic (study)

Ewing BB50 average number of occurrences per hour of the event between two successive R-to-R intervals exceeding 50 ms during a 24-hour period.

F French system of diameter measurement (as for a needle or catheter tip)

FM frequency modulation

FN false negative (algorithm verification rating)

FP false positive (algorithm verification rating)

FFT Fast-Fourier transform

F waves flutter waves

HP heart period

hr hour

HR heart rate

HRV heart rate variability

HZ (or Hz) Hertz; measure of frequency

ICD implantable cardioverter-defibrillator

ISO isolation circuitry signal path

JET junctional ectopic tachycardia

LAS low amplitude signal

Leads

   I bipolar lead on two wrists

   II bipolar lead on right wrist and two ankles

   III bipolar lead on left wrist and two ankles

   MCL_1 modified bipolar lead placed under the outer aspect of the right clavicle

   aVF augmented limb lead

   aVL augmented left limb lead

   aVR augmented right limb lead

   Ebp esophageal lead

   V_1-V_6 the six unipolar precordial leads

   V_1R unipolar precordial lead at the fourth intercostal space at the right margin of the sternum

   V_2R unipolar precordial lead at the fourth intercostal space at the left margin of the sternum

   V_3R unipolar precordial lead midway between sites V_2 and V_4

   V_4R unipolar precordial lead at the fifth intercostal space at the midclavicular line

   V_5R unipolar precordial lead at the same level of V_4 at the anterior axillary line

   V_6R unipolar precordial lead at the same level of V_4 at the midaxillary line

V$_7$	unipolar precordial lead at the posterior axial line		SCA	sudden cardiac arrest
V$_8$	unipolar precordial lead at the angle of the scapula		SCD	sudden cardiac death
			SD	standard deviation
V$_9$	unipolar precordial lead over the spine		SDANN	standard deviation of the means of successive 5-minute blocks of heart rate measurements over 24 hours.

V$_7$ unipolar precordial lead at the posterior axial line

V$_8$ unipolar precordial lead at the angle of the scapula

V$_9$ unipolar precordial lead over the spine

X lead placed in the fourth intercostal space in both midaxillary lines

XYZ the three orthogonal leads

Y lead placed on the superior aspect of the manubrium and the upper left leg or left iliac crest

Z lead placed on the left side of the vertebral column

LP late potential

MAT multifocal atrial tachycardia

MI (or mi) myocardial infarction (heart attack)

min minute

mm millimeter

ms millisecond

MUX multiplexed; operation digitizing XYZ lead signals on an ECG

mV millivolt

μV microvolt

NS normal sinus

n(t) accompanying noise in ECG signal

occ/hour number of occurrences per hour

PAC premature atrial complex

pi (π) correlation coefficient

PJC premature junctional complex

PJRT permanent junctional reciprocating tachycardia

pNNSD percent of absolute differences between successive normal beats that exceed 50 ms

PVC premature ventricular contraction

R (beats) the number of beats

√R square root of the number of beats averaged

RMS40 amplitude of the terminal 40 msecs

RMSSD a measure of the variation of changes in R-to-R interval length from one beat to the next.

RSA respiratory sinus arrhythmia

s$_1$ signal component of each beat

SCA sudden cardiac arrest

SCD sudden cardiac death

SD standard deviation

SDANN standard deviation of the means of successive 5-minute blocks of heart rate measurements over 24 hours.

SDIndex Magid Statistic (or AVESTD); average of SDs of successive 5-minute blocks of heart rate measurements over 24 hours.

sec second

SIDS sudden infant death syndrome

s$_i$(t) signal component of each beat

SNR signal-to-noise ratio

s(t) cardiac signal component

STM spectrotemporal mapping

SV supraventricular

SVT supraventricular tachycardia

T time resolution

TP true positive (algorithm verification rating)

VCG vectorcardiogram

VF ventricular fibrillation

VM(t) vector magnitude waveform

VT ventricular tachycardia

Waves

QRS the first downward deflection, plus the first upward deflection, plus the first downward deflection following the R wave on the ECG recording

R the first upward deflection on the ECG recording

ST-T the portion of the ECG signal extending from the end of the QRS complex to the beginning of the T wave; usually flat or slightly inclined.

T the portion of the ECG signal occurring during ventricular repolarization, hyperventilation, or after ingesting hot or cold substances

WAP wandering atrial pacemaker

WPW Wolff-Parkinson-White (syndrome)

x(t) the measured ECG

XYZ the three orthogonal leads

10.0   REFERENCES

1. Einthoven W: The different forms of the human electrocardiogram and their signification. Lancet 1:853, 1912.

2. Wilson FN, Johnston FD, MacLeod AG, et al.: Electrocardiograms that represent the potential variations of a single electrode. Am Heart J 9:477, 1934.

3. Goldberger E: A simple, indifferent electrocardiographic electrode of zero potential and a technique of obtaining augmented, unipolar, extremity leads. Am Heart J 23:483, 1942.

4. Committee of the American Heart Association for the Standardization of Precordial Leads: Standardization of precordial leads. (a) Supplementary report. Am Heart J 15:235, 1938; (b) Second supplementary report. JAMA 121:1349, 1943.

5. Rawlings CA: Biophysical Measurement Series: Electrocardiography. Redmond, SpaceLabs, Inc., 1991.

6. Sendon JL, Coma-Canella I, Alcasena S, et al.: Electrocardiographic findings in acute right ventricular infarction: sensitivity and specificity of electrocardiographic alterations in right precordial leads V_4R,V_3R, V_1, V_2, and V_3. J Am Coll Cardiol 6:1273, 1985.

7. Nehb W: Zur Standardisierung der Brustwandableitungen des Elektrokardiogramms. Mit Bemerkungen zum Fruhbild des Hinterwandinfarkts und des Infarktnachschubs in der Vorderwand. Klin Wochenscher 17:1807, 1938.

8. Marriott HJL: Practical Electrocardiology. Eighth Edition. Baltimore, Williams and Wilkins, 1988.

9. Committee on Electrocardiography of The American Heart Association: Recommendations for standardization of leads and of specifications for instruments in electrocardiography and vectorcardiography. Circulation 52:11, 1975.

10. Fumagalli B: Unipolar value of standard limb leads: lead -aVR and rational arrangement of limb leads. Am Heart J 48:204, 1954.

11. Cabrera E: Electrocardiography Clinique: Theorie et Pratique. Paris, Mason, 1959.

12. Dower GE, Nazzal SB, Pahlm O, et al.: Limb leads of the electrocardiogram: sequencing revisited. Clin Cardiol 13:346, 1990.

13. Frank E: An accurate, clinically practical system for spatial vectorcardiography. Circulation 13:737, 1956.

14. Willems JL, Lesaffre E, Pardaens J: Comparison of the classification ability of the electrocardiogram and vectorcardiogram. Am J Cardiol 59:119, 1987.

15. McFee R, Parungao A: An orthogonal lead system for clinical electrocardiography. Am Heart J 62:93, 1961.

16. Macfarlane PW, Lorimer AR, Lawrie TDV: 3 and 12 lead electrocardiogram interpretation by computer. A comparison of 1093 patients. Br Heart J 33:266, 1971.

17. Macfarlane PW: A Hybrid Lead System for Routine Electrocardiography. In: Progress in Electrocardiology. Macfarlane PW (Ed). Tunbridge Wells, Pitman Medical, 1979.

18. Castellanos A, Sung RJ, Richter S, et al.: XYZ electrocardiography. Correlation with conventional 12-lead electrocardiogram. Cardiovasc Clin 3:285, 1977.

19. Marriott HJL, Fogg E: Constant monitoring for dysrhythmias and blocks. Mod Concepts Cardiovasc Dis 39:103, 1970.

20. Mason RE, Likar I: A new system of multiple-lead exercise electrocardiography. Am Heart J 71:196, 1966.

21. American College of Cardiology Task Force II: Quality of electrocardiographic records. Am J Cardiol 41:146, 1965.

22. Sevilla DC, Dohrmann ML, Somelofski CA, et al.: Invalidation of the resting electrocardiogram obtained via exercise electrode sites as a standard 12-lead recording. Am J Cardiol 63:45, 1989.

23. Edenbrandt L, Pahlm O, Sormo L: An accurate exercise lead system for bicycle ergometer tests. Curr Heart J 10:268, 1989.

24. Pahlm O, Haisty Jr WK, Edenbrandt L, et al.: Evaluation of changes in standard electrocardiographic QRS waveforms recorded from activity compatible proximal lead positions. Am J Cardiol, In press, 1992.

25. Froelicher Jr VF, Wolthins R, Keiser N, et al.: A comparison of two exercise electrocardiographic leads to lead V_5. Chest 70:611, 1976.

26. Miller TD, Desser KB, Lawson M: How many electrocardiographic leads are required for exercise treadmill testing? J Electrocardiol 20:131, 1987.

27. van Dam TR, Corstens FJM, Uijen GJH, et al.: Correlation between ST-60 surface maps and TI-201 scintigrams in exercise induced myocardial ischemia. J Electrocardiol 24:284, 1991.

28. The Task Force of the Committee on Electro-cardiography and Cardiac Electrophysiology of the Council on Clinical Cardiology: Recommendations for standards of instrumentation and practice in the use of ambulatory electrocardiography. Circulation 71:626A, 1985.

29. MacAlpin RN: Correlation of the location of coronary artery spasm with the lead distribution of ST segment elevation during variant angina. Am Heart J 99:555, 1980.

30. Tanabe T, Yoshioka K, Kitada M, et al.: Evaluation of a newly devised three-lead Holter recording during treadmill testing in the diagnosis of ischemic ST changes. J Electrocardiol 24:155, 1991.

31. Schnittger I, Rodriguez IM, Winkle RA: A new technology revives an old technique. Am J Cardiol 57:604, 1986.

32. Krucoff MW, Pope JE, Bottner RK, et al.: Computer-assisted ST segment monitoring: experience during and after brief coronary occlusion. J Electrocardiol 20 (Suppl):15, 1987.

33. Taccardi B: Body surface mapping and cardiac electric sources. J Electrocardiol 23 (Suppl):150, 1990.

34. Fox KM, Deanfield J, Ribero P, et al.: Projection of ST segment changes onto the front of the chest; Practical implications for exercise testing and ambulatory monitoring. Br Heart J 48:555, 1982.

35. Lux RL: Mapping Techniques. In: Comprehensive Electrocardiography - Theory and Practice. Macfarlane PW, Lawrie TDV (Eds). New York, Permagon Press, 1989.

36. Ambroggi LD, Negroni MS, Monza E, et al.: Dispersion of ventricular repolarization in the long QT syndrome. Am J Cardiol 68:614, 1991.

37. Baule GM, McFee R: Detection of the magnetic field of the heart. Am Heart J 66:95, 1963.

38. Simson M: Use of signals in the terminal QRS complex to identify patients with ventricular tachycardia after myocardial infarction. Circulation 64:235, 1981.

39. Faugère G, Savard P, Nadeau RA, et al.: Characterization of the spatial distribution of late ventricular potentials by body surface mapping in patients with ventricular tachycardia. Circulation 74:1323, 1986.

40. Task Force Committee of the European Society of Cardiology, the American Heart Association, and the American College of Cardiology: Standards for analysis of ventricular late potentials using high-resolution or signal-averaged electrocardiography. Circulation 83:1481, 1991.

41. Atwood E, Myers J, Forbes S, et al.: High-frequency electrocardiography: an evaluation of lead placement and measurement. Am Heart J 116:733, 1988.

42. Huiskamp GJ, van Oosterom A: Influence of heart position and orientation on the inversely calculated ventricular activation sequence. J Electrocardiol 24:290, 1991.

43. Dower GE, Bastos Machado H: Progress report on the ECG. In: Progress in Electrocardiography. Macfarlane PW (Ed). Tunbridge Wells, Pitman Medical, 1979.

44. Chou T: When is the vectorcardiogram superior to the scaler electrocardiogram? Circulation 8:781, 1986.

45. Hurd HP, Starling MR, Crawford MH, et al.: Comparative accuracy of electrocardiographic and vectorcardiographic criteria for inferior infarction. Circulation 63:1025, 1981.

46. Warner R, Hill NE, Sheehe PR, et al.: Improved electrocardiographic criteria for the diagnosis of inferior myocardial infarction. Circulation 66:422, 1982.

47. Edenbrandt L, Pahlm O: Vectorcardiogram synthesized from a 12-lead ECG: superiority of the inverse Dower matrix. J Electrocardiol 21:361, 1988.

48. Kors JA, van Herpen G, Sittig AC, et al.: Reconstruction of the Frank vectorcardiogram from standard electrocardiographic leads: diagnostic comparison of different methods. Eur Heart J 11:1083, 1990.

49. Stallmann FW, Pipberger HV: Automatic recognition of electrocardiographic waves by digital computer. Circ Res 9:1138, 1961.

50. Pipberger HV: Computer analysis of the electrocardiogram. In: Computers in Biomedical Research. Stacy RW, Waxman B (Eds). New York, Academic Press, 1965.

51. Golden DP, Wolthuis RA, Hoffler GW: A spectral analysis of the normal resting electrocardiogram. IEEE Trans Biomed Engineer BME 20:366, 1973.

52. Cox JR, Nolle FM, Fozzard HA, et al.: AZTEC, a preprocessing program for real-time ECG rhythm analysis. IEEE Trans Biomed Engineer BME 15:128, 1968.

53. Pan J, Tompkins WJ: A real-time QRS detection algorithm. IEEE Trans Biomed Engineer BME 32:230, 1985.

54. Nygards ME, Hulting J: Recognition of ventricular fibrillation from the power spectrum of the ECG. Computers in Cardiology, New York, IEEE Press, 1977.

55. Aubert AE, Goldreyer BN, Wyman MG, et al.: Recognition of ventricular fibrillation and tachycardia from electrogram analysis. Computers in Cardiology, New York, IEEE Press, 1988.

56. Hermes RE, Arthur RM, Thomas Jr LJ, et al.: Status of the American Heart Association Database. Computers in Cardiology, New York, IEEE Press, 1979.

57. Mark RG, Schluter PS, Moody GB, et al.: An annotated ECG database for evaluating arrhythmia detectors. In: Frontiers of Engineering in Health Care. New York, IEEE Engineering in Medicine and Biology Society, 1982.

58. Association for the Advancement of Medical Instrumentation: Testing and reporting performance results of ventricular arrhythmia detection algorithms. AAMI recommended practice. Arlington, AAMI, 1987.

59. Abildskov JA: The sequence of normal recovery of excitability in the dog heart. Circulation 52:442, 1975.

60. Marcus ML: The Coronary Circulation in Health and Disease. New York, McGraw Hill, 1983.

61. Samson WE, Scher AM: Mechanism of ST segment alteration during acute myocardial injury. Circ Res 8:780, 1960.

62. Mirvis DM, Berson AS, Goldberger AL, et al.: Instrumentation and practice standards for electrocardiographic monitoring in special care units. Circulation 79:464, 1989.

63. Sheffield LT, Berson A, Bragg-Remschel D, et al.: Recommendations for standards of instrumentation and practice in the use of ambulatory electrocardiography. Circulation 71:636A, 1985.

64. Mason RE, Likar I: A new system of multiple-lead exercise electrocardiography. Am Heart J 71:196, 1966.

65. Association for Advancement of Medical Instrumentation: American National Standard, Cardiac Monitors, Heart Rate Meters and Alarms (ANSI/AAMI EC13-1983). Arlington, Association for the Advancement of Medical Instrumentation, 1984.

66. Tayler D, Vincent R: Signal distortion in the electrocardiogram due to inadequate phase response. IEEE Trans Biomed Engineer BME 30:352, 1983.

67. Pipberger HV, Arzbaecher RC, Berson AS, et al.: American Heart Association Committee on Electrocardiography: Recommendations for standardization of leads and of specifications for instruments in electrocardiography and vectorcardiography. Circulation 52:11, 1975.

68. Rocco MB, Nabel EG, Campbell S, et al.: Prognostic importance of myocardial ischemia detected by ambulatory monitoring in patients with stable coronary artery disease. Circulation 78:877, 1988.

69. Rocco MB, Barry J, Campbell S, et al.: Circadian variation of transient myocardial ischemia in patients with coronary artery disease. Circulation 75:395, 1987.

70. Selwyn AP: Current technology in assessing painless and painful ischemia. Am Heart J 120:722, 1990.

71. Deanfield JE, Shea M, Ribiero P, et al.: Transient ST segment depression as a marker of myocardial ischemia during daily life. Am J Cardiol 54:1195, 1984.

72. Deedwania PC, Nelson JR: Pathophysiology of silent myocardial ischemia during daily life. Hemodynamic evaluation by simultaneous electrocardiographic and blood pressure monitoring. Circulation 82:1296, 1990.

73. Droste C, Roskamm H: Experimental pain measurement in patients with asymptomatic myocardial ischemia. J Am Coll Cardiol 1:940, 1983.

74. Carboni GP, Lahiri A, Cashman PMM, et al.: Mechanisms of arrhythmias accompanying ST segment depression on ambulatory monitoring in stable angina pectoris. Am J Cardiol 60:1246, 1987.

75. Tzivoni D, Weisz G, Gavish A, et al.: Comparison of mortality and myocardial infarction rates in stable angina pectoris with and without ischemic episodes during daily activities. Am J Cardiol 63:273, 1989.

76. Nademanee K, Intarachot V, Josephson MA, et al.: Prognostic significance of silent myocardial ischemia in patients with unstable angina. J Am Coll Cardiol 10:1, 1987.

77. Ouyang P, Chandra NC, Gottlieb SO: Frequency and importance of silent myocardial ischemia identified with ambulatory electrocardiographic monitoring in the early in-hospital period after acute myocardial infarction. Am J Cardiol 65:267, 1990.

78. Tzivoni D, Gavish A, Zin D, et al.: Prognostic significance of ischemic episodes in patients with previous myocardial infarction. Am J Cardiol 62:661, 1988.

79. Mangano DT, Browner WS, Hollenberg M, et al.: Association of perioperative myocardial ischemia with cardiac morbidity and mortality in men undergoing noncardiac surgery. N Engl J Med 323:1781, 1990.

80. Garson Jr A, Bricker JT, McNamara DG (Eds): The Science and Practice of Pediatric Cardiology. Philadelphia, Lea & Febiger, 1990.

81. Anderson RA, Macartney F, Shinebourne EA, et al. (Eds): Pediatric Cardiology. Edinburgh, Churchill Livingstone, 1987.

82. Adams FH, Emmanouilides GC, Riemenschneider TA (Eds): Moss' Heart Disease in Infants, Children and Adolescents. Baltimore, Williams and Wilkins, 1989.

83. Kleinman CS, Copel JA, Weinstein EM, et al.: In utero diagnosis and treatment of fetal supraventricular tachycardia. Semin Perinatol 9:113, 1985.

84. Klapholz H: Techniques of fetal heart rate monitoring. Semin Perinatol 2:119, 1978.

85. Wheeler T, Murrills A, Shelly T: Measurement of the fetal heart rate during pregnancy by a new electrocardiographic technique. Br J Obstet Gynaecol 85:12, 1978.

86. Perry JC, McQuinn RC, Smith Jr RT, et al.: Flecainide acetate for resistant arrhythmias in the young: efficacy and pharmacokinetics. J Am Coll Cardiol 14:185, 1989.

87. Houyel L, Fournier A, Davignon A: Successful treatment of chaotic atrial tachycardia with oral flecainide. Intl J Cardiol 27:27, 1990.

88. Esscher E, Michaelsson M: QT interval in congenital complete heart block. Pediatr Cardiol 4:121, 1983.

89. Taylor PV, Scott JS, Gerlis LM, et al.: Maternal antibodies against fetal cardiac antigens in congenital complete heart block. N Engl J Med 315:667, 1986.

90. Perry JC, Garson Jr A: Supraventricular tachycardia due to Wolff-Parkinson-White syndrome in children: early disappearance and late recurrence. J Am Coll Cardiol 16:1215, 1990.

91. Villain E, Vetter VL, Garcia JM, et al.: Evolving concepts in the management of congenital junctional ectopic tachycardia. A multicenter study. Circulation 81:1544, 1990.

92. Coumel P, Cabrol C, Fabiato A, et al.: Tachycardie permanente par rhythm reciproque. Arch Mal Coeur 60:1830, 1967.

93. Critelli G, Gallagher JJ, Monda V, et al.: Anatomic and electrophysiologic substrate of the permanent form of junctional reciprocating tachycardia. J Am Coll Cardiol 4:601, 1984.

94. Gallagher JJ, Sealy WC: The permanent form of junctional reciprocating tachycardia: further elucidation of the underlying mechanism. Eur J Cardiol 8:413, 1978.

95. O'Neill BJ, Klein GJ, Guiraudon GM, et al.: Results of operative therapy in the permanent form of junctional reciprocating tachycardia. Am J Cardiol 63:1074, 1989.

96. Kuck KH, Geiger M, Schluter M, et al.: Radiofrequency current catheter ablation of accessory pathways in children. J Am Coll Cardiol 17:292A, 1991.

97. Garson Jr A, Smith Jr RT, Moak JP, et al.: Incessant ventricular tachycardia in infants: myocardial hamartomas and surgical cure. J Am Coll Cardiol 10:619, 1987.

98. Chandar JS, Wolff GS, Garson Jr A, et al.: Ventricular arrhythmias in postoperative tetralogy of Fallot. Am J Cardiol 65:655, 1990.

99. Garson Jr A, Randall DC, Gillette PC, et al.: Prevention of sudden death after repair of tetralogy of Fallot: treatment of ventricular arrhythmias. J Am Coll Cardiol 6:221, 1985.

100. Garson Jr A, Smith Jr RT, Moak JP, et al.: Ventricular arrhythmias and sudden death in children. J Am Coll Cardiol 5:130B, 1985.

101. Scagliotti D, Strasburg B, Duffy CE, et al.: Inducible polymorphous ventricular tachycardia following Mustard operation for transposition of the great arteries. Pediatr Cardiol 5:39, 1984.

102. Kugler JD, Danford DA: Pacemakers in children: an update. Am Heart J 117:665, 1989.

103. Smith Jr RT: Pacemakers for bradycardia. In: The Science and Practice of Pediatric Cardiology. Garson Jr A, Bricker JT, McNamara DG (Eds). Philadelphia, Lea & Febiger, 1990.

104. Frye RL, Collins JJ, DeSanctis RW, et al.: Guidelines for permanent cardiac pacemaker implantation. J Am Coll Cardiol 4:434, 1984.

105. Graham FK, Jackson JC: Arousal systems and infant heart rate responses. In: Advances in Child Development and Behavior. Reese HW, Lipsitt LP (Eds). New York, Academic Press, Volume 5, 1970.

106. Khachaturian ZS, Kerr J, Kruger R, et al.: A methodological comparison of period and rate data in studies of cardiac function. Psychophysiology 9:539, 1972.

107. Jennings JR, Stringfellow JC, Graham M: A comparison of the statistical distributions of beat-by-beat heart rate and heart period. Psychophysiology 14:89, 1974.

108. Graham FK: Normality of distributions and homogeneity of variance of heart rate and heart period samples. Psychophysiology 15:487, 1974.

109. Graham FK: Constraints on measuring heart rate and period sequentially through real and cardiac time. Psychophysiology 15:492, 1978.

110. Kleiger R, Miller J, Bigger J, et al.: Decreased heart rate variability and its association with increased mortality after acute myocardial infarction. Am J Cardiol 59:256, 1987.

111. Magid NM, Martin G, Kehoe RF, et al.: Diminished heart rate variability in sudden cardiac death. Circulation 72 (Suppl):241, 1985.

112. Martin G, Magid N, Valentini V, et al.: Heart rate variability and the evaluation of the risk of sudden cardiac death. Clin Res 35:203, 1987.

113. Martin GJ, Magid N, Ekberg D, et al.: Heart rate variability and sudden cardiac death during ambulatory monitoring. Clin Res 35:302a, 1987.

114. Kleiger RE, Miller J, Bigger Jr JT, et al.: Heart rate variability: a variable predicting mortality following acute myocardial infarction. J Am Coll Cardiol 59:547, 1984.

115. Ewing DJ, Neilson J, Travis P: New method for assessing cardiac parasympathetic activity using 24-hour electrocardiograms. Br Heart J 52:396, 1984.

116. Bigger JT, Albrecht P, Steinman RC, et al.: Comparison of time and frequency domain-based measures of cardiac parasympathetic activity in Holter recordings after myocardial infarction. Am J Cardiol 64:536, 1989.

117. Bigger JT, Kleiger R, Rolintzky LP, et al.: Components of heart rate variability measured during healing of acute myocardial infarction. Am J Cardiol 61:208, 1988.

118. Myers GA, Martin G, Magid MN, et al.: Power spectral analysis of heart rate variability in sudden cardiac death: comparison to other methods. IEEE Trans Biomed Engineer BME 12:1149, 1986.

119. Porges S: The application of spectral analysis for the detection of fetal distress. In: Infants Born at Risk. Fields, Sostek, Goldberg, et al. (Eds). New York, Spectrum, 1979.

120. Porges S, Arnold W, Forbes E: Heart rate variability: an index of attentional responsivity in human newborns. Dev Psychology 3:85, 1973.

121. Kitney RI, Rompelman O: The Study of Heart Rate Variability. Oxford, Clarendon Press, 1980.

122. Shin S, Tapp W, Reisman S, et al.: Assessment of autonomic regulation of heart rate variability by the method of complex demodulation. IEEE Trans Biomed Engineer BME 2:274, 1989.

123. Gordon D, Cohen R, Kelly D, et al.: Sudden infant death syndrome: abnormalities in short term fluctuations in heart rate and respiratory activity. Pediatr Res 18:921, 1984.

124. Harris FJ: On the use of windows for harmonic analysis with the Discrete-Fourier transform. Proc IEEE 66:51, 1978.

125. Bendat JS, Piersol AG: Random Data: Analysis and Measurement Procedures. New York, Wiley-Interscience, 1971.

126. Baselli G, Cerutti S, Civardi S, et al.: Heart rate variability signal processing: a quantitative approach as an aid to diagnosis in cardiovascular pathologies. Intl J Biomed Computing 20:51, 1987.

127. Lisenby MJ, Richardson PC: The Beatquency domain: an unusual application of the Fast-Fourier transform. IEEE Trans Biomed Engineer BME 24:4, 1977.

128. Cowan MJ, Kogan HN, Burr R, et al.: Power spectral analysis of heart rate variability after biofeedback training. J Electrocardiol 23 (Suppl):85, 1991.

129. Goldberger AL, Rigney D, West B: Chaos and fractals in human physiology. Sci Am 262:43, 1990.

130. Goldberger AL, Rigney D, Mietus J, et al.: Nonlinear dynamics in sudden cardiac death syndrome: heart rate oscillations and bifurcations. Experientia 44:983, 1988.

131. Theiler J: Estimating fractal dimension. J Opt Soc Am A 7:1055, 1990.

132. Pritchard WS, Duke D: Dimensional analysis of the human EEG using the Grassberger-Procaccia method. Technical report FSU-SCRI-90-115, Tallahassee, Florida State University, 1990.

133. Pritchard WS, Duke D, Coburn K: Dimensional analysis of topographic EEG: some methodological considerations. Technical Report FSU-SCRI-90T-146, Tallahassee, Florida State University, 1990.

134. Rapp PE, Bashore TR, Martinerie JM, et al.: Dynamics of brain electrical activity. Brain Topogr 2:99, 1989.

135. Rapp PE, Albano A, Mees A: Calculation of correlation dimensions from experimental data: progress and problems. In: Dynamic Patterns in Complex Systems. Kelso JAS, Mandell AJ, Schlesinger M (Eds). Singapore, World Scientific, 1988.

136. Lo PC, Principle JC: Dimensionality analysis: experimental considerations. Proc Int Conf Neural Networks, 1989.

137. Grassberger P, Procaccia I: Measuring the strangeness of strange attractors. Physica D 9:189, 1983.

138. Bassingthwaite JB, van Beek J: Lightning and the heart: fractal behavior in cardiac function. Proc IEEE 76:693, 1988.

139. Mayer-Kress G, Yates FE, Benton L, et al.: Dimensional analysis of nonlinear oscillations in brain, heart, and muscle. Math Biosci 90:155, 1988.

140. Bekheit S, Tangella M, el Sakr A, et al.: Use of heart rate spectral analysis to study the effects of calcium channel blockers on sympathetic activity after myocardial infarction. Am Heart J 119:79, 1990.

141. Vybiral T, Bryg R, Maddens ME, et al.: Effects of transdermal scopolamine on heart rate variability in normal subjects. Am J Cardiol 65:604, 1990.

142. Berbari EJ, Lazzara R, Samet P, et al.: Noninvasive technique for detection of electrical activity during the P-R segment. Circulation 48:1005, 1973.

143. Scherlag BJ, Lau SH, Helfant RH, et al.: Catheter technique for recording His bundle activity in man. Circulation 39:13, 1969.

144. El-Sherif N, Scherlag BJ, Lazzara R, et al.: Re-entrant ventricular arrhythmias in the late myocardial infarction period. In: Conduction characteristics in the infarctionzone. Circulation 55:686, 1977.

145. Berbari EJ, Lazzara R: An introduction to high-resolution ECG recordings of cardiac late potentials. Arch Intern Med 148:1859, 1988.

146. Tompkins WJ, Webster JG: Design on Microcomputer-Based Medical Instrumentation. Englewood Cliffs, Prentice Hall Inc., 1981.

147. Bragg-Remschel DA, Anderson CM, Winkle RA: Frequency response characteristics of ambulatory ECG monitoring systems and their implications on ST segment analysis. Am Heart J 111:103, 1982.

148. Rompelman O, Ros HH: Coherent averaging technique: a tutorial review. Part 2: Trigger jitter, overlapping responses and non-periodic stimulation. J Biomed Engineer 8:30, 1986.

149. Jané R, Rix H, Caminal P, et al.: Alignment methods for averaging of high-resolution cardiac signals: a comparative study of performance. IEEE Trans Biomed Engineer 38:571, 1991.

150. Rompelman O, Ros HH: Coherent averaging technique: a tutorial review. Part 1: Noise reduction and the equivalent filter. J Biomed Engineer 8:24, 1986.

151. Steinberg JS, Bigger JT: Importance of the endpoint of noise reduction in analysis of the signal-averaged electrocardiogram. Am J Cardiol 63:556, 1989.

152. Lander P, Berbari EJ, Rajagopalan CV, et al.: Critical analysis of the signal-averaged electrocardiogram: improved identification of late potentials. Circulation, Submitted 1992.

153. Lander P, Berbari EJ: Optimizing signal averaging methods. IEEE Engr Med Bio Soc 11th Annual Int'l Conf, 11-A:19, 1989.

154. Lander P, Berbari EJ: Use of highpass filtering to detect late potentials in the signal-averaged ECG. J Electrocardiol 225:7, 1989.

155. Simson MB: Use of signals in the terminal QRS complex to identify patients with ventricular tachycardia after myocardial infarction. Circulation 64:235, 1981.

156. Lander P, Deal RB, Berbari EJ: The analysis of ventricular late potentials using orthogonal recordings. IEEE Trans Biomed Engineer BME 35:629, 1988.

157. Berbari EJ: High resolution electrocardiography. CRC Crit Rev Biomed Engr 16:67, 1988.

158. Pietersen AH, Gymoese E, Breithardt G: Importance of the noise level for detection of late potentials in the signal-averaged electrocardiogram. Circulation 82:711, 1990.

159. Cain ME, Ambos HD, Witkowski FX, et al.: Fast-Fourier transform analysis of signal-averaged electrocardiograms for identification of patients prone to sustained ventricular tachycardia. Circulation 69:711, 1984.

160. Lander P, Albert DE, Berbari EJ: Spectrotemporal analysis of ventricular late potentials. J Electrocardiol 23:95, 1990.

161. Haberl R, Schels HF, Steinbigler P, et al.: Top-resolution frequency analysis of electrocardiogram with adaptive frequency determination. Circulation 82:1183, 1990.

162. Lander P, Berbari EJ: Spectral analysis of the high resolution ECG as an equivalent filter problem. J Electrocardiol 24:21, 1992.

11.0   ILLUSTRATION CREDITS

Figure 3.8

Cox JR, Noelle FM: AZTEC, a processing program for real time EKG rhythm analysis. IEEE Trans Biomed Engineer BME 2:128, 1968.

Figure 4.5

Mason RE, Likar I: A new system of multiple-lead exercise electrocardiography. American Heart J 71:196, 1966.

Figure **4.6**

Kennedy H: Ambulatory Electrocardiography. Philadelphia, Lea & Febiger, 1981.

Figure 4.8

Selwyn AP: Current technology in assessing painless and painful ischemia. American Heart J 120:722, 1990.

Figure 6.5

Kleiger R, Miller J, Bigger J, et al.: Decreased heart rate variability and its association with increased mortality after acute myocardial infarction. Am J Cardiol 59:256, 1987.

Figure 6.8

Myers GA, Martin G, Magid NM, et al.: Power spectral analysis of heart rate variability in sudden cardiac death: comparison to other methods. IEEE Trans Biomed Engineer BME 33:1149, 1986.

Figure 6.9

Basselli G, Cerutti S, Civardi S, et al.: Heart rate variability signal processing: A quantitative approach as an aid to diagnosis in cardiovascular pathologies. Int J Biomed Computing 20:51, 1987.

Figure 6.12

Lisenby M, Richardson P: The beatquency domain: an unusual application of the Fast-Fourier transform. IEEE Trans Biomed Engineer BME 24:4, 1977.

12.0 BIBLIOGRAPHY

The following bibliograpahy lists, in chronologic order, citations pertinent to the study of electrocardiography.

12.1 Lead Systems

Einthoven W: The different forms of the human electrocardiogram and their signification. Lancet 1:853, 1912.

Wilson FN, Johnston FD, MacLeod AG, et al.: Electrocardiograms that represent the potential variations of a single electrode. Am Heart J 9:477, 1934.

Nehb W: Zur Standardisierung der Brustwandableitungen des Elektrokardiogramms. Mit Bemerkungen zum Fruhbild des Hinterwandinfarkts und des Infarkt-nachschubs in der Vorderwand. Klin Wochenscher 17:1807, 1938.

Goldberger E: A simple, indifferent electrocardiographic electrode of zero potential and a technique of obtaining augmented, unipolar, extremity leads. Am Heart J 23:483, 1942.

Committee of the American Heart Association for the Standardization of Precordial Leads: Standardization of precordial leads. (a) Supplementary report. Am Heart J 15:235, 1938; (b) Second supplementary report. JAMA 121:1349, 1943.

Fumagalli B: Unipolar value of standard limb leads: lead -aVR and rational arrangement of limb leads. Am Heart J 48:204, 1954.

Frank E: An accurate, clinically practical system for spatial vectorcardiography. Circulation 13:737, 1956.

Cabrera E: Electrocardiography Clinique: Theorie et Pratique. Paris, Mason, 1959.

McFee R, Parungao A: An orthogonal lead system for clinical electrocardiography. Am Heart J 62:93, 1961.

Baule GM, McFee R: Detection of the magnetic field of the heart. Am Heart J 66:95, 1963.

American College of Cardiology Task Force II: Quality of electrocardiographic records. Am J Cardiol 41:146, 1965.

Mason RE, Likar I: A new system of multiple-lead exercise electrocardiography. Am Heart J 71:196, 1966.

Marriott HJL, Fogg E: Constant monitoring for dysrhythmias and blocks. Mod Concepts Cardiovasc Dis 39:103, 1970.

Macfarlane PW, Lorimer AR, Lawrie TDV: 3 and 12 lead electrocardiogram interpretation by computer. A comparison of 1093 patients. Br Heart J 33:266, 1971.

Committee on Electrocardiography of The American Heart Association: Recommendations for standardization of leads and of specifications for instruments in electrocardiography and vectorcardiography. Circulation 52:11, 1975.

Froelicher Jr VF, Wolthins R, Keiser N, et al.: A comparison of two exercise electrocardiographic leads to lead V5. Chest 70:611, 1976.

Castellanos A, Sung RJ, Richter S, et al.: XYZ electrocardiography. Correlation with conventional 12 lead electrocardiogram. Cardiovasc Clin 3:285, 1977.

Macfarlane PW: A Hybrid Lead System for Routine Electrocardiography. In: Progress in Electrocardiology. Macfarlane PW (Ed). Tunbridge Wells, Pitman Medical, 1979.

Dower GE, Bastos Machado H: Progress report on the ECG. In: Progress in Electrocardiography. Macfarlane PW (Ed). Tunbridge Wells, Pitman Medical, 1979.

MacAlpin RN: Correlation of the location of coronary artery spasm with the lead distribution of ST segment elevation during variant angina. Am Heart J 99:555, 1980.

Simson M: Use of signals in the terminal QRS complex to identify patients with ventricular tachycardia after myocardial infarction. Circulation 64:235, 1981.

Hurd HP, Starling MR, Crawford MH, et al.: Comparative accuracy of electrocardiographic and vectorcardiographic criteria for inferior infarction. Circulation 63:1025, 1981.

Fox KM, Deanfield J, Ribero P, et al.: Projection of ST segment changes onto the front of the chest; Practical implications for exercise testing and ambulatory monitoring. Br Heart J 48:555, 1982.

Warner R, Hill NE, Sheehe PR, et al.: Improved electrocardiographic criteria for the diagnosis of inferior myocardial infarction. Circulation 66:422, 1982.

Sendon JL, Coma-Canella I, Alcasena S, et al.: Electrocardiographic findings in acute right-ventricular infarction: sensitivity and specificity of electrocardiographic alterations in right precordial leads V_4R, V_3R, V_1, V_2, and V_3. J Am Coll Cardiol 6:1273, 1985.

The Task Force of the Committee on Electrocardiography and Cardiac Electrophysiology of the Council on Clinical Cardiology: Recommendations for standards of instrumentation and practice in the use of ambulatory electrocardiography. Circulation 71:626A, 1985.

Schnittger I, Rodriguez IM, Winkle RA: A new technology revives an old technique. Am J Cardiol 57:604, 1986.

Faugère G, Savard P, Nadeau RA, et al.: Characterization of the spatial distribution of late ventricular potentials by body surface mapping in patients with ventricular tachycardia. Circulation 74:1323, 1986.

Chou T: When is the vectorcardiogram superior to the scaler electrocardiogram? Circulation 8:781, 1986.

Willems JL, Lesaffre E, Pardaens J: Comparison of the classification ability of the electrocardiogram and vectorcardiogram. Am J Cardiol 59:119, 1987.

Miller TD, Desser KB, Lawson M: How many electrocardiographic leads are required for exercise treadmill testing? J Electrocardiol 20:131, 1987.

Krucoff MW, Pope JE, Bottner RK, et al.: Computer-assisted ST segment monitoring: experience during and after brief coronary occlusion. J Electrocardiol 20 (Suppl):15, 1987.

Marriott HJL: Practical Electrocardiology. Eighth Edition. Baltimore, Williams and Wilkins, 1988.

Atwood E, Myers J, Forbes S, et al.: High-frequency electrocardiography: an evaluation of lead placement and measurement. Am Heart J 116:733, 1988.

Edenbrandt L, Pahlm O: Vectorcardiogram synthesized from a 12-lead ECG: superiority of the inverse Dower matrix. J Electrocardiol 21:361, 1988.

Sevilla DC, Dohrmann ML, Somelofski CA, et al.: Invalidation of the resting electrocardiogram obtained via exercise electrode sites as a standard 12-lead recording. Am J Cardiol 63:45, 1989.

Edenbrandt L, Pahlm O, Sormo L: An accurate exercise lead system for bicycle ergometer tests. Curr Heart J 10:268, 1989.

Lux RL: Mapping Techniques. In: Comprehensive Electrocardiography - Theory and Practice. Macfarlane PW, Lawrie TDV (Eds). New York, Permagon Press, 1989.

Dower GE, Nazzal SB, Pahlm O, et al.: Limb leads of the electrocardiogram: sequencing revisited. Clin Cardiol 13:346, 1990.

Taccardi B: Body surface mapping and cardiac electric sources. J Electrocardiol 23 (Suppl):150, 1990.

Kors JA, van Herpen G, Sittig AC, et al.: Reconstruction of the Frank vectorcardiogram from standard electrocardiographic leads: diagnostic comparison of different methods. Eur Heart J 11:1083, 1990.

van Dam TR, Corstens FJM, Uijen GJH, et al.: Correlation between ST-60 surface maps and TI-201 scintigrams in exercise induced myocardial ischemia. J Electrocardiol 24:284, 1991.

Tanabe T, Yoshioka K, Kitada M, et al.: Evaluation of a newly devised three-lead Holter recording during treadmill testing in the diagnosis of ischemic ST changes. J Electrocardiol 24:155, 1991.

Ambroggi LD, Negroni MS, Monza E, et al.: Dispersion of ventricular repolarization in the long QT syndrome. Am J Cardiol 68:614, 1991.

Task Force Committee of the European Society of Cardiology, the American Heart Association, and the American College of Cardiology: Standards for analysis of ventricular late potentials using high-resolution or signal-averaged electrocardiography. Circulation 83:1481, 1991.

Rawlings CA: Biophysical Measurement Series: Electrocardiography. Redmond, SpaceLabs, Inc., 1991.

Huiskamp GJ, van Oosterom A: Influence of heart position and orientation on the inversely calculated ventricular activation sequence. J Electrocardiol 24:290, 1991.

Pahlm O, Haisty Jr WK, Edenbrandt L, et al.: Evaluation of changes in standard electrocardiographic QRS waveforms recorded from activity-compatible proximal lead positions. Am J Cardiol, In press, 1992.

12.2 Electrical Physiology of the Heart

Huszar R: Basic Disrhythmias - Interpretation and Management. St. Louis, CV Mosby Co., 1988.

Davis D: How to Quickly and Accurately Master Arryhthmia Interpretation. Philadelphia, JB Lippincott, 1989.

Jacobson C: Basic arrhythmias and conduction disturbances. In: Cardiac Nursing. Underhill, Woods, Froelicher, et al. (Eds). Philadelphia, JB Lippincott, 1989.

Marriott HJL, Conover M: Advanced Concepts in Arrhythmias. 2nd Ed. St. Louis, CV Mosby Co., 1989.

Patel J, McGowan S., Moody L: Arrhythmias: Detection, Treatment, and Cardiac Drugs. Philadelphia, WB Saunders Co., 1989.

Atwood S, Stanton C, Storey J: Introduction to Basic Cardiac Dysrhythmias. St. Louis, CV Mosby Co., 1990.

Phillips R, Feeney M: The Cardiac Rhythms: A Systematic Approach to Interpretation. 3rd Ed. Philadelphia, WB Saunders Co., 1990.

12.3 Arrythmia Detection Algorithms

Stallmann FW, Pipberger HV: Automatic recognition of electrocardiographic waves by digital computer. Circ Res 9:1138, 1961.

Pipberger HV: Computer analysis of the electrocardiogram. In: Computers in Biomedical Research. Stacy RW, Waxman B (Eds). New York, Academic Press, 1965.

Cox JR, Nolle FM, Fozzard HA, et al.: AZTEC, a preprocessing program for real-time ECG rhythm analysis. IEEE Trans Biomed Engineer BME 15:128, 1968.

Golden DP, Wolthuis RA, Hoffler GW: A spectral analysis of the normal resting electrocardiogram. IEEE Trans Biomed Engineer BME 20:366, 1973.

Nygards ME, Hulting J: Recognition of ventricular fibrillation from the power spectrum of the ECG. Computers in Cardiology, New York, IEEE Press, 1977.

Hermes RE, Arthur RM, Thomas Jr LJ, et al.: Status of the American Heart Association Database. Computers in Cardiology, New York, IEEE Press, 1979.

Mark RG, Schluter PS, Moody GB, et al.: An annotated ECG database for evaluating arrhythmia detectors. In: Frontiers of Engineering in Health Care. New York, IEEE Engineering in Medicine and Biology Society, 1982.

Pan J, Tompkins WJ: A real-time QRS detection algorithm. IEEE Trans Biomed Engineer BME 32:230, 1985.

Association for the Advancement of Medical Instrumentation: Testing and reporting performance results of ventricular arrhythmia detection algorithms. AAMI recommended practice. Arlington, AAMI, 1987.

Aubert AE, Goldreyer BN, Wyman MG, et al.: Recognition of ventricular fibrillation and tachycardia from electrogram analysis. Computers in Cardiology, New York, IEEE Press, 1988.

12.4 ST Segment Analysis

Samson WE, Scher AM: Mechanism of ST segment alteration during acute myocardial injury. Circ Res 8:780, 1960.

Mason RE, Likar I: A new system of multiple-lead exercise electrocardiography. Am Heart J 71:196, 1966.

Abildskov JA: The sequence of normal recovery of excitability in the dog heart. Circulation 52:442, 1975.

Pipberger HV, Arzbaecher RC, Berson AS, et al.: American Heart Association Committee on Electrocardiography: Recommendations for standardization of leads and of specifications for instruments in electrocardiography and vectorcardiography. Circulation 52:11, 1975.

Marcus ML: The Coronary Circulation in Health and Disease. New York, McGraw Hill, 1983.

Tayler D, Vincent R: Signal distortion in the electrocardiogram due to inadequate phase response. IEEE Trans Biomed Engineer BME 30:352, 1983.

Droste C, Roskamm H: Experimental pain measurement in patients with asymptomatic myocardial ischemia. J Am Coll Cardiol 1:940, 1983.

Association for Advancement of Medical Instrumentation: American National Standard, Cardiac Monitors, Heart Rate Meters and Alarms (ANSI/ AAMI EC13-1983). Arlington, Association for the Advancement of Medical Instrumentation, 1984.

Deanfield JE, Shea M, Ribiero P, et al.: Transient ST segment depression as a marker of myocardial ischemia during daily life. Am J Cardiol 54:1195, 1984.

Sheffield LT, Berson A, Bragg-Remschel D, et al.: Recommendations for standards of instrumentation and practice in the use of ambulatory electrocardiography. Circulation 71:636A, 1985.

Rocco MB, Barry J, Campbell S, et al.: Circadian variation of transient myocardial ischemia in patients with coronary artery disease. Circulation 75:395, 1987.

Nademanee K, Intarachot V, Josephson MA, et al.: Prognostic significance of silent myocardial ischemia in patients with unstable angina. J Am Coll Cardiol 10:1, 1987.

Carboni GP, Lahiri A, Cashman PMM, et al.: Mechanisms of arrhythmias accompanying ST segment depression on ambulatory monitoring in stable angina pectoris. Am J Cardiol 60:1246, 1987.

Rocco MB, Nabel EG, Campbell S, et al.: Prognostic importance of myocardial ischemia detected by ambulatory monitoring in patients with stable coronary artery disease. Circulation 78:877, 1988.

Tzivoni D, Gavish A, Zin D, et al.: Prognostic significance of ischemic episodes in patients with previous myocardial infarction. Am J Cardiol 62:661, 1988.

Mirvis DM, Berson AS, Goldberger AL, et al.: Instrumentation and practice standards for electrocardiographic monitoring in special care units. Circulation 79:464, 1989.

Tzivoni D, Weisz G, Gavish A, et al.: Comparison of mortality and myocardial infarction rates in stable angina pectoris with and without ischemic episodes during daily activities. Am J Cardiol 63:273, 1989.

Selwyn AP: Current technology in assessing painless and painful ischemia. Am Heart J 120:722, 1990.

Deedwania PC, Nelson JR: Pathophysiology of silent myocardial ischemia during daily life. Hemodynamic evaluation by simultaneous electrocardiographic and blood pressure monitoring. Circulation 82:1296, 1990.

Ouyang P, Chandra NC, Gottlieb SO: Frequency and importance of silent myocardial ischemia identified with ambulatory electrocardiographic monitoring in the early in-hospital period after acute myocardial infarction. Am J Cardiol 65:267, 1990.

Mangano DT, Browner WS, Hollenberg M, et al.: Association of perioperative myocardial ischemia with cardiac morbidity and mortality in men undergoing noncardiac surgery. N Engl J Med 323:1781, 1990.

12.5 Pediatric Electrocardiography

Coumel P, Cabrol C, Fabiato A, et al.: Tachycardie permanente par rhythm reciproque. Arch Mal Coeur 60:1830, 1967.

Klapholz H: Techniques of fetal heart rate monitoring. Semin Perinatol 2:119, 1978.

Wheeler T, Murrills A, Shelly T: Measurement of the fetal heart rate during pregnancy by a new electrocardiographic technique. Br J Obstet Gynaecol 85:12, 1978.

Gallagher JJ, Sealy WC: The permanent form of junctional reciprocating tachycardia: further elucidation of the underlying mechanism. Eur J Cardiol 8:413, 1978.

Esscher E, Michaelsson M: QT interval in congenital complete heart block. Pediatr Cardiol 4:121, 1983.

Critelli G, Gallagher JJ, Monda V, et al.: Anatomic and electrophysiologic substrate of the permanent form of junctional reciprocating tachycardia. J Am Coll Cardiol 4:601, 1984.

Scagliotti D, Strasburg B, Duffy CE, et al.: Inducible polymorphous ventricular tachycardia following Mustard operation for transposition of the great arteries. Pediatr Cardiol 5:39, 1984.

Frye RL, Collins JJ, DeSanctis RW, et al.: Guidelines for permanent cardiac pacemaker implantation. J Am Coll Cardiol 4:434, May 1984.

Kleinman CS, Copel JA, Weinstein EM, et al.: In utero diagnosis and treatment of fetal supraventricular tachycardia. Semin Perinatol 9:113, 1985.

Garson Jr A, Randall DC, Gillette PC, et al.: Prevention of sudden death after repair of tetralogy of Fallot: treatment of ventricular arrhythmias. J Am Coll Cardiol 6:221, 1985.

Garson Jr A, Smith Jr RT, Moak JP, et al.: Ventricular arrhythmias and sudden death in children. J Am Coll Cardiol 5:130B, 1985.

Taylor PV, Scott JS, Gerlis LM, et al.: Maternal antibodies against fetal cardiac antigens in congenital complete heart block. N Engl J Med 315:667, 1986.

Anderson RA, Macartney F, Shinebourne EA, et al. (Eds): Pediatric Cardiology. Edinburgh, Churchill Livingstone, 1987.

Garson Jr A, Smith Jr RT, Moak JP, et al.: Incessant ventricular tachycardia in infants: myocardial hamartomas and surgical cure. J Am Coll Cardiol 10:619, 1987.

Adams FH, Emmanouilides GC, Riemenschneider TA (Eds): Moss' Heart Disease in Infants, Children and Adolescents. Baltimore, Williams and Wilkins, 1989.

Perry JC, McQuinn RC, Smith Jr RT, et al.: Flecainide acetate for resistant arrhythmias in the young: efficacy and pharmacokinetics. J Am Coll Cardiol 14:185, 1989.

O'Neill BJ, Klein GJ, Guiraudon GM, et al.: Results of operative therapy in the permanent form of junctional reciprocating tachycardia. Am J Cardiol 63:1074, 1989.

Kugler JD, Danford DA: Pacemakers in children: an update. Am Heart J 117:665, 1989.

Garson Jr A, Bricker JT, McNamara DG (Eds): The Science and Practice of Pediatric Cardiology. Philadelphia, Lea & Febiger, 1990.

Houyel L, Fournier A, Davignon A: Successful treatment of chaotic atrial tachycardia with oral flecainide. Intl J Cardiol 27:27, 1990.

Perry JC, Garson Jr A: Supraventricular tachycardia due to Wolff-Parkinson-White syndrome in children: early disappearance and late recurrence. J Am Coll Cardiol 16:1215, 1990.

Villain E, Vetter VL, Garcia JM, et al.: Evolving concepts in the management of congenital junctional ectopic tachycardia. A multicenter study. Circulation 81:1544, 1990.

Chandar JS, Wolff GS, Garson Jr A, et al.: Ventricular arrhythmias in postoperative tetralogy of Fallot. Am J Cardiol 65:655, 1990.

Smith Jr RT: Pacemakers for bradycardia. In: The Science and Practice of Pediatric Cardiology. Garson Jr A, Bricker JT, McNamara DG (Eds). Philadelphia, Lea & Febiger, 1990.

Kuck KH, Geiger M, Schluter M, et al.: Radiofrequency current catheter ablation of accessory pathways in children. J Am Coll Cardiol 17:292A, 1991.

12.6 Heart Rate Variability

Graham FK, Jackson JC: Arousal systems and infant heart rate responses. In: Advances in Child Development and Behavior. Reese HW, Lipsitt LP (Eds). New York, Academic Press, Volume 5, 1970.

Bendat JS, Piersol AG: Random Data: Analysis and Measurement Procedures. New York, Wiley-Interscience, 1971.

Khachaturian ZS, Kerr J, Kruger R, et al.: A methodological comparison of period and rate data in studies of cardiac function. Psychophysiology 9:539, 1972.

Porges S, Arnold W, Forbes E: Heart rate variability: an index of attentional responsivity in human newborns. Dev Psychology 3:85, 1973.

Jennings JR, Stringfellow JC, Graham M: A comparison of the statistical distributions of beat-by-beat heart rate and heart period. Psychophysiology 14:89, 1974.

Graham FK: Normality of distributions and homogeneity of variance of heart rate and heart period samples. Psychophysiology 15:487, 1974.

Lisenby MJ, Richardson PC: The Beatquency domain: an unusual application of the Fast-Fourier transform. IEEE Trans Biomed Engineer BME 24:4, 1977.

Graham FK: Constraints on measuring heart rate and period sequentially through real and cardiac time. Psychophysiology 15:492, 1978.

Harris FJ: On the use of windows for harmonic analysis with the Discrete-Fourier transform. Proc IEEE 66:51, 1978.

Porges S: The application of spectral analysis for the detection of fetal distress. In: Infants Born at Risk. Fields, Sostek, Goldberg, et al. (Eds). New York, Spectrum, 1979.

Kitney RI, Rompelman O: The Study of Heart Rate Variability. Oxford, Clarendon Press, 1980.

Grassberger P, Procaccia I: Measuring the strangeness of strange attractors. Physica D 9:189, 1983.

Kleiger RE, Miller J, Biggers Jr JT, et al.: Heart rate variability: a variable predicting mortality following acute myocardial infarction. J Am Coll Cardiol 59:547, 1984.

Ewing DJ, Neilson J, Travis P: New method for assessing cardiac parasympathetic activity using 24-hour electrocardiograms. Br Heart J 52:396, 1984.

Gordon D, Cohen R, Kelly D, et al.: Sudden infant death syndrome: abnormalities in short term fluctuations in heart rate and respiratory activity. Pediatr Res 18:921, 1984.

Magid NM, Martin G, Kehoe RF, et al.: Diminished heart rate variability in sudden cardiac death. Circulation 72 (Suppl):241, 1985.

Myers GA, Martin G, Magid MN, et al.: Power spectral analysis of heart rate variability in sudden cardiac death: comparison to other methods. IEEE Trans Biomed Engineer BME 12:1149, 1986.

Kleiger R, Miller J, Bigger J, Moss A: Decreased heart rate variability and its association with increased mortality after acute myocardial infarction. Am J Cardiol 59:256, 1987.

Martin GJ, Magid N, Valentini V, et al.: Heart rate variability and the evaluation of the risk of sudden cardiac death. Clin Res 35:203, 1987.

Martin GJ, Magid N, Ekberg D, et al.: Heart rate variability and sudden cardiac death during ambulatory monitoring. Clin Res 35:302a, 1987.

Baselli G, Cerutti S, Civardi S, et al.: Heart rate variability signal processing: a quantitative approach as an aid to diagnosis in cardiovascular pathologies. Intl J Biomed Computing 20:51, 1987.

Bigger JT, Kleiger R, Rolintzky LP, et al.: Components of heart rate variability measured during healing of acute myocardial infarction. Am J Cardiol 61:208, 1988.

Goldberger AL, Rigney D, Mietus J, et al.: Nonlinear dynamics in sudden cardiac death syndrome: heart rate oscillations and bifurcations. Experientia 44:983, 1988.

Rapp PE, Albano A, Mees A: Calculation of correlation dimensions from experimental data: progress and problems. In: Dynamic Patterns in Complex Systems. Kelso JAS, Mandell AJ, Schlesinger M (Eds). Singapore, World Scientific, 1988.

Bassingthwaite JB, van Beek J: Lightning and the heart: fractal behavior in cardiac function. Proc IEEE 76:693, 1988.

Mayer-Kress G, Yates FE, Benton L, et al.: Dimensional analysis of nonlinear oscillations in brain, heart, and muscle. Math Biosci 90:155, 1988.

Bigger JT, Albrecht P, Steinman RC, et al.: Comparison of time and frequency domain-based measures of cardiac parasympathetic activity in Holter recordings after myocardial infarction. Am J Cardiol 64:536, 1989.

Shin S, Tapp W, Reisman S, et al.: Assessment of autonomic regulation of heart rate variability by the method of complex demodulation. IEEE Trans Biomed Engineer BME 2:274, 1989.

Rapp PE, Bashore TR, Martinerie JM, et al.: Dynamics of brain electrical activity. Brain Topography 2:99, 1989.

Lo PC, Principle JC: Dimensionality analysis: experimental considerations. Proc Int Conf Neural Networks, 1989.

Goldberger AL, Rigney D, West B: Chaos and fractals in human physiology. Sci Am 262:43, 1990.

Theiler J: Estimating fractal dimension. J Opt Soc Am A 7:1055, 1990.

Pritchard WS, Duke D: Dimensional analysis of the human EEG using the Grassberger-Procaccia method. Technical report FSU-SCRI-90-115, Tallahassee, Florida State University, 1990.

Pritchard WS, Duke D, Coburn K: Dimensional analysis of topographic EEG: some methodological considerations. Technical Report FSU-SCRI-90T-146, Tallahassee, Florida State University, 1990.

Bekheit S, Tangella M, el Sakr A, et al.: Use of heart rate spectral analysis to study the effects of calcium channel blockers on sympathetic activity after myocardial infarction. Am Heart J 119:79, 1990.

Vybiral T, Bryg R, Maddens ME, et al.: Effects of transdermal scopolamine on heart rate variability in normal subjects. Am J Cardiol 65:604, 1990.

Cowan MJ, Kogan HN, Burr R, et al.: Power spectral analysis of heart rate variability after biofeedback training. J Electrocardiol 23 (Suppl):85, 1991.

12.7 Late Potentials and the Electrocardiogram

Scherlag BJ, Lau SH, Helfant RH, et al.: Catheter technique for recording His bundle activity in man. Circulation 39:13, 1969.

Berbari EJ, Lazzara R, Samet P, et al.: Noninvasive technique for detection of electrical activity during the P-R segment. Circulation 48:1005, 1973.

El-Sherif N, Scherlag BJ, Lazzara R, et al.: Re-entrant ventricular arrhythmias in the late-myocardial infarction period. In: Conduction characteristics in the infarction zone. Circulation 55:686, 1977.

Tompkins WJ, Webster JG: Design on Microcomputer-Based Medical Instrumentation. Englewood Cliffs, Prentice Hall Inc., 1981.

Simson MB: Use of signals in the terminal QRS complex to identify patients with ventricular tachycardia after myocardial infarction. Circulation 64:235, 1981.

Bragg-Remschel DA, Anderson CM, Winkle RA: Frequency response characteristics of ambulatory ECG monitoring systems and their implications on ST segment analysis. Am Heart J 111:103, 1982.

Cain ME, Ambos HD, Witkowski FX, et al.: Fast-Fourier transform analysis of signal-averaged electrocardiograms for identification of patients prone to sustained ventricular tachycardia. Circulation 69:711, 1984.

Rompelman O, Ros HH: Coherent averaging technique: a tutorial review. Part 2: Trigger jitter, overlapping responses and non-periodic stimulation. J Biomed Engineer 8:30, 1986.

Rompelman O, Ros HH: Coherent averaging technique: a tutorial review. Part 1: Noise reduction and the equivalent filter. J Biomed Engineer 8:24, 1986.

Berbari EJ, Lazzara R: An introduction to high-resolution ECG recordings of cardiac late potentials. Arch Intern Med 148:1859, 1988.

Lander P, Deal RB, Berbari EJ: The analysis of ventricular late potentials using orthogonal recordings. IEEE Trans Biomed Engineer BME 35:629, 1988.

Berbari EJ: High resolution electrocardiography. CRC Crit Rev Biomed Engr 16:67, 1988.

Steinberg JS, Bigger JT: Importance of the endpoint of noise reduction in analysis of the signal-averaged electrocardiogram. Am J Cardiol 63:556, 1989.

Lander P, Berbari EJ: Optimizing signal averaging methods. IEEE Engr Med & Bio Soc 11th Annual Int'l Conf, 11-A:19, 1989.

Lander P, Berbari EJ: Use of highpass filtering to detect late potentials in the signal-averaged ECG. J Electrocardiol 225:7, 1989.

Pietersen AH, Gymoese E, Breithardt G: Importance of the noise level for detection of late potentials in the signal-averaged electrocardiogram. Circulation 82:711, 1990.

Lander P, Albert DE, Berbari EJ: Spectrotemporal analysis of ventricular late potentials. J Electrocardiol 23:95, 1990.

Haberl R, Schels HF, Steinbigler P, et al.: Top-resolution frequency analysis of electrocardiogram with adaptive frequency determination. Circulation 82:1183, 1990.

Jané R, Rix H, Caminal P, et al.: Alignment methods for averaging of high-resolution cardiac signals: a comparative study of performance. IEEE Trans Biomed Engineer 38:571, 1991.

Lander P, Berbari EJ: Spectral analysis of the high resolution ECG as an equivalent filter problem. J Electrocardiol 24:21, 1992.

Lander P, Berbari EJ, Rajagopalan CV, et al.: Critical analysis of the signal-averaged electrocardiogram: improved identification of late potentials. Circulation, submitted 1992.

13.0   GLOSSARY

Accelerated ventricular rhythm — The rhythm of the beats of the ventricles of the heart that are faster than the normal rhythms; occurs when an ectopic focus in the ventricles fires at a rate of 50 to 100 beats per minute.

Action potential — The varying difference in electric potential across the membrane of an active cell.

Acute myocardial infarction (AMI) — A sudden heart attack; a blockage of any of the essential blood vessels that provide oxygen to the heart muscle.

Algorithm — A mathematical computational procedure.

Algorithm verification — A test or series of tests to verify or prove the computational worth of a procedure.

Ambulatory monitoring, 24-hour — The 24-hour electrocardiographic monitoring of patient who is connected to a measurement instrument during daily activities.

Amplitude-Zone-Time-Epoch-Coding (AZTEC) — A preprocessor for electrocardiographic signals; an algorithm that compresses high sampling rate information into a series of straight line segments that can then be processed by later algorithm stages in an effectively much lower sampling rate.

Antegrade — Moving or extending forward.

Arrhythmia — Any irregularity in the force of the heartbeat.

Atria — Plural of atrium (see atrium).

Atrial arrhythmia — The irregular rhythm of contraction or firing of the atrium of the heart.

Atrial fibrillation — The extremely rapid and disorganized pattern of the depolarization of the atria.

Atrial flutter — The extremely rapid depolarization of the atria at rates of 250 to 350 times per minute.

Atrial lead — Another name for the bipolar precordial lead, usually placed to the right of the sternum.

Atrial myocarditis — Inflammation of the myocardial tissue of the atrium of the heart.

Atrial tachycardia — The rapid atrial rhythm occurring at a rate of 150 to 250 bpm; when arrhythmia starts and stops abruptly, it is called "paroxysmal atrial tachycardia".

Atrioventricular node (AV node) — A mass of specialized cells in the right atrium, medial to the right atrioventricular valve and continuous with the other atrial cells and with the atrioventricular bundle; often divided by electrophysiologists into three functional regions: the atrio-nodal (AN), the nodal (N), and the nodal-His (NH).

Atrioventricular block — Arrhythmias in which delayed or failed conduction of the supraventricular impulses into the ventricles occur.

Atrium — In anatomy, a chamber allowing entrance to another structure or organ; in cardiac anatomy, one of the two upper chambers of the heart.

Augmented leads — Leads used in electrocardiography that are added to increase the signals recorded and the information received during the recording.

Automatic implantable cardioverter-defibrillator (AICD) — A device that detects ventricular fibrillation and tachycardia from electrodes implanted in the myocardium and processes it using mathematical algorithms.

Automaticity — The ability of certain parts of the heart to initiate an impulse without an external stimulus.

AV block — The blockage of the atrioventricular node.

AV junction — The junction of the atrium and the ventricle of the heart.

AV node — See atrioventricular node.

Baseline wander — A drifting in the recording of a signal; random and slow deviations from the reference line of a signal recorded with respect to time.

Beatquency — Cycles per heart beat.

Beat detection — Recording of the type and frequency of the heartbeat.

Biplane fluoroscopy — A technique that measures the instantaneous localization of the catheter position used for electrophysiologic studies in pediatric patients.

Bipolar lead — A lead that acts by means of two poles.

Bipolar precordial lead — A lead that acts by means of two poles that are placed over the precordium, the region of the body over the heart or stomach (includes the epigastrium and the lower part of the thorax).

Body surface mapping — A map of the equipotential contours of the body determined by measurements at many locations on the skin, usually on the chest and back.

Bradycardia — An abnormal heart rate of 60 or fewer bpm.

Bundle of His — A small band of atypical cardiac muscle fibers that originate in the atrioventricular node in the right atrium and pass through the endocardium to the right ventricle on the membranous part of the interventricular septum; propagates the atrial contraction rhythm to the ventricles.

Central autonomic nervous system (CANS) — The section of the nervous system responsible for many of the "automatic" responses of the body such as organ function and hormone secretion.

Chaotic atrial tachycardia — An infantile arrhythmia occurring at atrial rates of 200 to 500 bpm; can include atrial tachycardia, flutter, and fibrillation.

Circadian rhythm — A periodicity of approximately 24 hours.

Congenital cardiac defects — Defects in the heart tissue present at birth.

Coronary artery obstruction — A blockage of the coronary artery that limits blood flow and seriously reduces the health of heart tissue.

Defibrillation — The application of direct current shock without synchronization; used during cardiac surgery to convert rhythms that are too fast or too erratic to synchronized rhythms.

Depolarization — The electrical excitation of the heart resulting from the flow of ions across the membrane of cardiac cells, which then spreads from cell to cell as a signal for contraction of the muscle tissue.

Dextrocardia — The positioning of the heart in the right side of the chest cavity with the apex of the heart pointing to the right.

Digital signal processor (DSP) — An integrated circuit chip used to measure Fast-Fourier transform.

Discrete-Fourier transform (DFT) — The heart period sequence or an estimate of its autocovariance function.

Doppler echocardiography — The measurement of heart parameters using Doppler ultrasound concepts; can be used to diagnose fetal arrhythmias.

ECG reconstruction — The reconstruction of the electrocardiogram from electrical or digital signal recordings.

Echocardiography — The medical discipline that measures the electrical signals from the heart to diagnose heart disease or obtain data regarding cardiac health.

Electrocardiogram (ECG, EKG) — The signal traced by an electrocardiograph; used in diagnosing heart disease or cardiac problems that modify the electrical activity of the heart.

Electrocardiography — The set of procedures that measure the electrical activity of the heart and record it on an electrocardiogram.

Electrode — An electric conductor through which a current enters or leaves a substance in contact with this device.

Electrode contact noise — Noise produced by the contact of an electrode with the skin.

Exercise testing — The assessment of a person's cardiac health, including measurement of ECG signals, during exercise, which usually comprises performance on a bicycle or treadmill.

False negative (FN) — The result of a measurement that produces a negative response although the actual response should be positive; an event occurred and was not correctly detected by a device.

False positive (FP) — The result of a measurement that indicates a positive response although the actual response should be negative; an event did not occur but was recorded by a device.

Fast-Fourier transform (FFT) — A mathematical procedure used to analyze periodic waves; the determination of the constant term and the coefficient of each term in the infinite series of waves including the sine and cosine components of the signal.

Feature extraction algorithm — Also, cluster analysis; an arrhythmia detection algorithm that uses only features and not shapes to distinguish the dominant from the ectopic beats by finding clusters in the parameter space.

Fetal arrhythmias — Irregular rhythms of the heart in the fetus while in utero; may indicate problems with the fetus prior to birth.

Fetal bradycardia — A heart rate below 100 bpm.

First-degree AV block — Prolonged AV conduction time of supraventricular impulses into the ventricles.

Gluteal fold — The section of the body where the buttock joins the leg.

Heart rate — The number of heart beats per unit time; usually measured as beats per minute (bpm).

Heart rate variability (HRV) — The normal variability of the heart rate.

High-grade AV block — Occurs when two or more consecutive atrial impulses are blocked when the atrial rate is less than 135 bpm.

High-resolution electrocardiography — Also signal-averaged electrocardiography; used to measure ventricular late potentials with modified or hybrid orthogonal lead systems.

His electrogram — An ECG with the electrical catheter inserted to the atrioventricular (AV) node and the bundle of His.

Holter recordings — The standard two-channel continuous bipolar recordings of the electrical activity of the heart using specific placements for the various leads, which are recommended by the American Heart Association.

HP variability — The variability in heart period.

HR variability — The variability in heart rate.

Hybrid algorithm — A mixture of mathematical procedures used to assess information or recorded data.

Instantaneous heart rate — Also instantaneous HR; the discrete event corresponding to the beating of the heart; the equivalent bpm that would have been measured if that particular cardiac cycle rate had been maintained exactly throughout a full 60-second period.

Interbeat interval (IBI) — The distance between adjacent P waves that reflects as closely as possible the statistics of the firing of the sinoatrial pacemaker node.

Jitter — The formation of timing errors in the trigger point on a device.

Junctional arrhythmia — An irregular rhythm originating at the AV junction.

Junctional ectopic tachycardia (JET) — A congenital or acquired condition following surgery for congenital heart defects.

Junctional rhythm — An arrhythmia that occurs if the sinus node rate falls below the automatic rate of the AV junctional pacemakers.

Junctional tachycardia — Excessively fast heartbeats at the AV junction.

Kleiger Global Standard Deviation — The beat-weighted standard deviation of the set of all the heart periods (R-to-R intervals) in a 24-hour interval.

Late potential — A highly amplified and filtered electrocardiographic voltage, usually toward the end of, or after, the QRS complex.

Lead — Electrocardiographic type; a signal; in electricity, a wire or other conductive medium.

Magnetocardiography — Cardiographic measurements based on the principles of magnetism.

Midaxillary line — The midsection of the area where the arm joins the body.

Modified bipolar lead (MCL₁) — A bipolar lead that has a neutral, or ground, electrode placed under the outer aspect of the right clavicle, the positive electrode in the position of lead V_1, and the negative electrode near the left shoulder.

Multifocal atrial tachycardia (MAT) — The rapid firing of several ectopic atrial regions at a rate faster than 100 bpm.

Myocardial infarction — Also, heart attack; the toxic lack of oxygen to the heart tissue due to the blockage of blood flow into an area of the heart.

Myocardial ischemia — The condition of the heart muscle resulting from an insufficient supply of oxygen and other nutrients to meet the metabolic demands of the cardiac tissue.

Noise — Any disturbance that obscures a signal or reduces its clarity or quality.

Orthogonal planes — Pertaining to lines at right angles to each other.

Pacemaker spike detection — Recording of the firing spike of the heart's natural pacemaker, the SA node.

Palpitations — Any irregular, rapid pulsation of the heart.

Parasternal window — The region of the body that lies alongside the sternum.

Parasympathetic nervous system — The part of the autonomic nervous system originating in the central and back parts of the brain and in the lower part of the spinal cord that inhibits or opposes the physiological effects of the sympathetic nervous system; for example, it slows the heart and stimulates digestion.

Pediatric electrophysiology (EP) — Invasive procedures that measure the electophysiologic status of young children.

Permanent junctional reciprocating tachycardia (PJRT) — An incessant supraventricular tachycardia found in young children.

pNNSD — The percent of the absolute differences between successive normal heart beats that exceed 50 msec.

Polar cardiography — An information processing system that graphically displays the magnitude and direction of the heart vector in relation to time.

Premature atrial complex (PAC) — These premature beats occur when an irritable focus in the atria fires before the next sinus impulse is due.

Premature junctional complex (PJC) — An arrhythmia resulting from an irritable focus in the AV junction that fires before the next sinus impulse is due.

P wave — The portion of the electrocardiogram that measures atrial depolarization.

PR interval — The portion of the electrocardiogram between the P wave and the succeeding R wave.

Pulse plethysmography — A system of measuring the local blood volume waveform.

Purkinje fibers — The muscle fibers at the end of the specialized conductive system of the heart; the widespread group of fibers in the ventricular subendocardium.

Q wave — The first downward deflection on the QRS complex.

QRS wave — Also the QRS complex; the signal on the electrocardiogram that represents the ventricular depolarization and atrial repolarization of the heart.

QRS width — The width of the entire QRS wave as measured on the electrocardiogram.

QT interval — The measured length from the beginning of the QRS complex to the end of the T wave on an electrocardiogram; relates to the duration of the depolarization and repolarization of the ventricles of the heart.

R-to-R interval — The space between the apex of the amplitude of an R wave and that of a succeeding R wave.

Rate (heart) — The number of heartbeats per unit time.

Real-time — The actual time in which a physical event under study occurs.

Refractory period — The period of time in which no response can occur; for example, once the ventricle has contracted, it requires time to reorganize itself for the next contraction.

Repolarization — In physiology, the relocation of some cellular ions to re-establish the transmembrane voltage of the resting cell, with negative polarity at the inside of the membrane; in the heart, the return of the organ to its electrical resting state due to ion flow across the cardiac cell membrane.

Resistance — Opposition or counter-acting force; an impediment to blood flow throughout the system.

Respiration — The process of exchanging waste carbon dioxide for oxygen in the body; at the cellular level, the release and use of energy to accomplish cellular processes.

Respiratory sinus arrhythmia (RSA) — A particular patterned sequence of changes in the heart interbeat interval coupled in a complex way to the respiratory behavior.

Retrograde — Moving or extending backward.

RMSSD — A measure of the variation of changes in R-to-R interval length from one beat to the next.

Scapular apex — A portion of the scapula; the triangular bones forming the back of the shoulder that point downward.

SDANN — The complement of the Magid Statistic; the standard deviation of the means of successive 5-minute blocks over 24 hours.

Second-degree AV block — Type I and Type II; occurs when one atrial impulse at a time fails to be conducted to the ventricles.

Semiorthogonal system — A system of leads used in vectorcardiography that includes mutual perpendicular leads in three planes and that places resistors in the circuit to correct for the magnitude of the vectors.

Signal averaging — The process whereby electrocardiographic signals are averaged over a specific time period.

Signal-to-noise ratio (SNR) — A measurement of the number of signals with respect to the noise measured during a given period of time.

Sinus arrest — Occurs when sinus node automaticity is depressed and impulses do not occur when expected, which results in the absence of a P wave at the time it should occur.

Sinus arrhythmia — Occurs when the sinus node discharges irregularly, exhibiting a decrease in heart rate.

Sinus bradycardia — Occurs when the sinus node discharges at a rate slower than 60 bpm.

Sinus node — The sinoatrial node of the heart; a mass of cells in the right atrium near the entrance of the superior vena cava; often called the pacemaker of the heart because the electrical activity in this node normally initiates the process leading to contraction of the heart.

Sinus tachycardia — The increased beating in the sinoatrial nodal area of the heart, usually at a rate greater than 100 bpm.

Spectrotemporal mapping (STM) — A procedure measuring the variation in high-resolution ECG measurements; performed by sliding a fixed-length window across the ECG waveform in small time increments and computing a sequence of spectra.

ST-T wave — The part of the electrocardiographic signal that includes the ST segment from the end of the QRS complex and the following T wave.

Sudden cardiac arrest (SCA) — A stoppage of the proper functioning of the heart muscle; a heart attack.

Sudden infant death syndrome (SIDS) — The interruption of breathing in an infant that leads to death; also called "crib death"; usually occurs within the first year of life.

Supraventricular tachycardia (SVT) — The narrow QRS tachycardia that occurs when the exact mechanism for the tachycardia cannot be determined from the surface ECG; indicates that the rhythm originates above the bifurcation of the bundle of His and that the ventricles are depolarized via the normal His-Purkinje system.

Sympathetic nervous system — A part of the autonomic nervous system that readies the body for the expenditure of energy; responsible for the "flight or fight" readiness of the body; for example, constricts blood vessels and stops digestion.

Tachycardia — Also tachyrhythmia; a rapid heartbeat; often used to classify heart rates of 100 or more bpm.

Telemetry — The science and technology of automatic measurement and transmission of data by wire, radio, or other means from remote sources to a receiving station for recording and analysis.

Template match (correlation) algorithms — Algorithms that use shape or morphology to distinguish the dominant from the ectopic beats in an ECG signal.

Third-degree AV block — Also, complete block; the complete failure of conduction of all atrial impulses to the ventricles.

Threshold trigger — A waveform and/or lead system used to produce a dynamic threshold to detect QRS complexes in patients with arrhythmias.

TP segment — The portion of the ECG from the T wave, which records ventricular repolarization, to the next P wave, which records atrial depolarization.

Transmembrane resting potential — The potential across a cellular membrane at rest.

Transient ischemia — A temporary toxic lack of oxygen in a particular portion of the heart tissue due to obstruction of the blood supply.

Transmural ischemia — A toxic lack of oxygen in the heart tissue that spreads across the membranes of the heart chambers.

True positive (TP) — An event occurred and was accurately detected by a device.

Unipolar lead — A lead that acts by means of one pole.

Unipolar precordial lead — A lead that acts by means of one pole that is placed over the precordium, the region of the body over the heart or stomach (includes the epigastrium and the lower part of the thorax).

Vectorcardiogram (VCG) — The recorded display of information received from a vectorcardiographic study; see vectorcardiography.

Vectorcardiography — The study or generation of displays of elliptical forms or figures representing the projection of the movement of the positive end of the cardiac dipole onto different planes, usually during a specific portion of the electrocardiogram; measures electrical activity in the frontal, horizontal, and sagittal planes.

Vector magnitude waveform [VM(t)] — A single parameter for presenting the information gathered from recordings from the three orthogonal XYZ leads.

Ventricular asystole — The absence of any ventricular rhythm; no cardiac output occurs.

Ventricular fibrillation (VF) — The rapid, ineffective quivering of the ventricles; becomes fatal if not treated immediately.

Ventricular hypertrophy — A morbid enlargement of the ventricle of the heart.

Ventricular tachycardia (VT) — Three or more ventricular beats in a row occurring at a rate of 100 bpm or faster.

Wander — The variance of a signal from an established baseline.

Wandering atrial pacemaker (WAP) — Occurs when the site of the impulse formation wanders from the sinus node to other pacemakers in the atria or when the atria and the AV junction compete with each other for control of the heart.

Wenckebach — Type I second-degree AV block; a progressive increase in conduction times of consecutive atrial impulses into the ventricles until one impulse fails to conduct or is dropped.

Wolff-Parkinson-White syndrome (WPW) — Also pre-excitation syndrome; a concurrence of electrocardiographic signs of abnormality in the electrical activity of the heart; visible in electrocardiograms of some patients with paroxysmal tachycardia.

Xiphoid process — The lower end of the sternum that is shaped like a sword.

INDEX

Accelerated ventricular rhythm 33, 35, 55
Acute myocardia infarction (AMI) 65, 68, 86, 96, 109
Algorithms 41-59
   Ambulatory (Holter) 41, 42
   Arrhythmia detection 41-59
   Box-Counting algorithm 106
   Grassberger-Proccacia algorithm 106
   Heart rate variability (HRV) 43, 59
   Holter scanner arrhythmia 41, 42
   Late potential (LP) 17, 43
   Real-time 41, 42, 47, 57
   ST segment 43
   Takens-Ellner algorithm 106
   Telemetry 41, 42
   Verification of 57
      False negative 57
      False positive 57
      True positive 57
Amplifiers 64, 113, 135
   AC-coupled amplifiers 64
   DC-coupled amplifiers 64
Amplitude-Zone-Time-Epoch-Coding (AZTEC) 47
Arrhythmia(s) 21-40, 69, 75-83
   Atria, in 26-31
      Premature atrial complex (PAC) 26, 79
      Wandering atrial pacemaker (WAP) 27
   Detection algorithms 41-59
   Monitoring 41, 42, 57-59
      Improved noise rejection 59
      Multiple leads 57
      ST segment type 59
   P waves 23-40, 79
   PR interval 23-40
   Rate 23, 69
   Respiratory sinus arrhythmia (RSA) 87
   QRS complexes 23, 25
   QRS width 23
   Regularity 21
   Sinus node, in 23-26
Association for the Advancement
of Medical Instrumentation (AAMI) 57
Asystole, ventricular 33, 36, 42
Atria, of heart 26-31
   Fibrillation of 26, 30, 75
   Flutter in 29, 33, 83, 143
   Multifocal atrial tachycardia (MAT) 28
   Myocarditis, in infants 79
   Paroxysmal atrial tachycardia 29
   Premature atrial complex (PAC) 26, 79
   Tachycardia in 29, 33, 75
   Wandering atrial pacemaker (WAP) 27
Atrioventricular block (see AV block)
Atrioventricular node 21, 23, 27-31, 37-40, 79, 83, 134, 137, 141
   Ablation of 83, 134, 141
   Modification of 134
Automaticity, heart 21, 31, 81
AV blocks 39, 37-40, 75, 79
   Complete 40
   Congenital complete AV block (CCAVB) 79
   First-degree 37
   High grade 39, 75
   Second-degree 37-38

   Type I (Wenckebach) 37
   Type II 38
   Third-degree (complete block) 40
AVESTD (see Magid Statistic) 96
AV junction 31-33
   Arrhythmias 31
      Junctional 31-33, 81
      Junctional ectopic tachycardia (JET) 81
      Junctional rhythms 31, 32
      Junctional tachycardias 31-33, 81
      Premature junctional complexes 31
AV node 21, 23, 31-40, 79, 134, 137
Bandpass filters 117, 123, 127, 129
Baseline wander 44, 67, 113
Beat, heart 51
   Classification 51-53
      Cluster analysis 51, 53
      Correlation type 51
      Feature extraction (cluster analysis) algorithms 53
      Hybrid algorithms 53
      Temple match (correlation) algorithms 51
   Detection 51
   Digital signal processor (DSP) 51
   Feature extraction 53
   Frequency domain features 51
   Onset 43, 59
   QRS complexes 41, 42, 51, 59
   Rhythm analysis 53
   Threshold trigger 51
   Time domain features 51
Beatquency 99
Blackman-Harris function 133
   ST segment measure 133
Blood pressure 42, 59, 68, 71, 85, 89
Body surface mapping 13, 15
Box-Counting algorithm 106
Bradycardia 24, 79
   Fetal 75
   Newborn, in the 79
   Sinus node 24, 79
Bundle of His 23, 33, 37, 79, 137
CANS transfer characteristics 89
Cardiac arrest 98, 143
Cardiac mapping 134, 137
   Induced tachycardia 139
   Wolff-Parkinson-White syndrome 139
Cardiac pacing 83
Cardioversion 135, 143
Cardioverter-defibrillator 135, 143, 145
   Automatic implantable (AICD) 43
   Implantable (ICD) 143, 145
Chaotic atrial tachycardia 75
Circadian rhythm 93
Congenital complete AV block (CCAVB) 79
Congestive heart failure (CHF) 75, 86, 105
Defibrillation 135, 143
Depolarization, heart 21, 31, 143
   Antegrade 31
   Retrograde 31
Diabetics 68, 86
   Transient ST segment depression in 68

Digital sampling, of ECG signal 55, 113-115
Discrete-Fourier transform (DFT) 101
Doppler electrocardiography 75
Electrocardiogram 21, 113, 123
   High-resolution 121, 129
      Frequency domain analysis 129
      Time domain analysis 121
      Use of 111
   Leads 3, 7, 55, 141
   Bipolar precordial lead 7
   Reconstruction of 17, 19
   Semi-orthogonal lead(s), XYZ leads 7, 11
   Standard, 12-lead 3, 13
      Reconstruction of 17, 19
   Vector magnitude waveform 127
Electrocardiographic lead 3
Electrocardiography
   Body surface mapping 13, 15
   Exercise type 13, 17
   Filtration, of signal 111, 113, 123, 141
      Highpass filtering 111, 123, 141
      Lowpass filtering 111, 123
   High resolution 17, 111
   Holter type 15, 17, 87
   Hybrid orthogonal 11, 17
   Late potentials 17, 127
   Magnetocardiography 17
   Modified orthogonal 17
   Orthogonal lead type 7, 11
   Pediatric electrocardiography 69-86
   Polar 11
   Signal-averaged 17
Electrodes
   Contact noise 44
   Epicardial 7
   Head (H) 11
   Midaxillary line (A) 11
   Negative 13
      CC5 (chest) 13
      CH5 (head) 13
      CM5 (manubrium) 13
      CR5 (arm) 13
      CS5 (shoulder) 13
   Pin-to-pin noise 44
   Positive 13
   Spine (M) 11
   Sternum (E) 11
Electrogram(s)
   His electrogram 137
   Intracavitary 134, 137
   Programmed electrical stimulation 137
   Purkinje system 137
   Superior vena cava 137
   Surface 134, 137
Electrophysiology 83, 134-146
   Cardiac pacing, studies of 83
   Digital processing 135
   Equipment used in 135
   Intracavitary electrograms 134, 137
   Recording devices 135
   Single-plane fluoroscopy 135
   Stimulators, for cardiac pacing 135, 137
   Surface electrograms 134, 137
Emergency Care Research Institute (ECRI) 57
Epicardial electrodes 7
Equivalent frequency 99

Ewing BB50 97
Exercise testing 13
Fast-Fourier transform (FFT) 51, 133
Fibrillation 30, 55
   Atrial 30
   Ventricular 33, 35, 41, 55, 79, 135, 143, 145
Filtration, of ECG signal 111, 123
   Highpass filtering 111, 123, 141
   Lowpass filtering 111, 123
Fluoroscopy 85, 135, 137
Flutter
   Atrial 29, 33, 75, 83, 143
   Ventricular 33, 143
Fractal (or Hausdorff) dimension 106
Frequency domain analysis 129
   High-resolution ECG 129
Grassberger-Proccacia algorithm 106
Heart
   Arrhythmia 21-40, 69, 75-83
      Rate 23, 61, 69
      Regularity 21
   Beat
      Beat status 107
      Nonsinus beats 87, 106
      Sinoatrial node 89
      Sinus type 81, 83, 117
   Bundle of His 23, 33, 37, 79, 137
   Depolarization 21, 31, 91
   Electrical physiology 134
   Instantaneous period 89
   Normal sinus rhythm 23
   Purkinje fibers 23
   Period 87, 95-110
   Rate 23, 61, 69, 86-110
   Rate variability (HRV) 86
   Refractory period 21, 137
   Repolarization 21, 143
   Rhythms
      P waves 23-40, 73, 79
      PR interval 23-40
      QRS complexes 23-40
      QRS width 23-40
      Sinus node 23
   Sinus rhythm 23
Heart period, instantaneous 89
Heart rate variability (HRV) 43, 86-110
   Acute myocardial infarction (AMI) 86
   Beatquency 99
   Beat weighting of 87, 95
   Central autonomic nervous system (CANS) in 86
   Clinical environment, measure of 109
   Congestive heart failure (CHF) 86
   Equivalent frequency 99
   Interbeat interval sequence 91
   Measures of
      AVESTD 96
      Ewing BB50 97
      24-Hour Holter monitoring 87, 96
      Kleiger Global Standard Deviation 96
      Magid SDIndex 96
      Magid Statistic (AVESTD or the SDIndex) 96
      pNN50 97
      Root mean square of successive differences (RMSSD) 96
      SDANN 97
      SDIndex 96

Physiologic models, for analysis 86
    CANS transfer characteristics 89
    Interbeat interval (IBI) 91
    Pulse plethysmography 91
    Raw electrocardiograph waveform 91
    R-to-R intervals 86
    Respiratory sinus arrhythmia (RSA) 87
    R-to-R interval 86
    Spectral analysis 87, 101
    Sudden cardiac death (SCD) 86
    Sudden infant death syndrome (SIDS) 86
    Time conversion factors 95
    Time weighting of 87, 95
His bundle 23, 33, 37, 79, 137
Holter monitoring 15
    Continuous 15
    Feet electrodes in 15
    Intermittent 15
    Three-channel bipolar 15
    Two-channel continuous bipolar 15, 57
Interbeat interval (IBI) 87, 91
Ischemia 61, 63, 68
    Myocardial 61, 63, 68
    Transient 61, 68-69
Isolation circuitry 115

Jitter 118
Junctional 31
    Impulse 31
    Rhythm 31, 32
Junctional ectopic tachycardia (JET) 81

Kleiger Global Standard Deviation 96

Late potential (LP) monitoring 17, 43, 111, 119, 129
Leads
    Augmented limb 3
    Bipolar 3, 141
    Modified bipolar 13
        MCL_1 13
    Presentation 7
    Problems with 7
    Selection of 3, 55
    Unipolar 3
    Unipolar precordial lead 3
        I, II, III 3, 7, 45, 71, 81, 137
        V_1-V_6 .... 3, 77, 65, 71, 81, 137
        V_2 .... 3, 17, 19, 65
        V_2R 3
        V_3R 3, 71
        V_4R 3, 71
        V_7 .... 3, 71
        V_8 3
        V_9 3
        aVF 3, 7, 65
        aVL 3, 7
        aVR 3, 7
        X 7, 11, 17, 113
        Y 7, 11, 17, 113
        Z 7, 11, 17, 113
Low frequency wander 44

Magid SDIndex 96
Magid Statistic (AVESTD or the SDIndex) 96
Magnetocardiography 17
Monitoring 13, 47
    Ambulatory 15, 42, 65
    Bedside 13, 42, 59
    Computerized 41

Continuous 15
Dedicated arrhythmia systems 41, 42
Fixed 17
Heart rate variability (HRV) 43, 59
Holter type 15, 42
Late potential (LP) 17, 43
Real-time 41, 42, 47, 57
Rhythm disturbances, for 13
ST segment 19, 43, 59
Telemetry 41, 42
Multifocal atrial tachycardia (MAT) 28
Muscle artifact 44
Myocardial infarction 19, 61, 68-69, 86, 96, 109, 111
Myocardial ischemia 61, 63, 68
    Electrocardiographic effects 64
    QRS complex 61, 64, 67
    Recording electrocardiographic effects 65
        Amplifier systems 64, 67
        Analysis systems 67
        ECG lead systems 3, 65
        J point 13, 67
        Monitor systems 65, 67
        QRS complex 67
    TP segment 64
Myocarditis, atrial in infants 79

Noise 43
    Detection 45, 47
    Rejection 45, 47, 59
    Removal of 45
    Sources of 43
        Baseline wander 44, 67, 113, 115
        Electrode contact type 44
        Low frequency wander 44
        Muscle artifact 44
        Pin-to-pin 44
        Power line interference 43
        Residual 119, 121
        Single electrode 45

Orthogonal-lead electrocardiography 7, 11, 17
    Hybrid orthogonal 11, 17
    Modified orthogonal 13

Pacemaker 27, 55
    Spike detection 55
    Wandering atrial 27
Parasternal window 13
Pediatric electrocardiography 69-86
Pediatric electrophysiology 85
    Biplane fluoroscopy 85
    Electrode catheter manipulation 85
    Sedation for 85
    Tachyarrhythmias 75, 81, 85
Permanent junctional reciprocating tachycardia (PJRT) 81
Permanent pacing systems, in children 83
pNN50 statistic 97
Polar cardiography 11
Premature atrial complex (PAC) 26, 79
    In newborns 79
Premature junctional complexes (PCJ) 31
Premature ventricular complexes (PVC) 33, 41, 97
Programmed electrical stimulation, of heart 137
Pulse plethysmography 91
Purkinje fibers 23
P wave 23-40, 59, 73, 79-111, 127
    Detection of 41, 59
    Monitoring of 41
QRS complex(es) 23-40, 41, 51, 59, 111, 123, 127, 143

Vector magnitude waveform 127
    Low amplitude signal (LAS) 127
    QRS duration 127, 129
    QRS offset 123, 127, 129
    QRS onset 123, 127, 129
    RMS40 .... 127, 129

Radiofrequency catheter ablation 83, 134, 141
Raw electrocardiograph waveform 91
Respiration 42, 44, 67, 89, 91, 118
Respiratory sinus arrhythmia (RSA) 87
Rhythm(s)
    Accelerated ventricular 35
    Normal 23
    P waves 23-40, 73, 79
    PR interval 23-40
    QRS complexes 23-40
    QRS width 23-40
    Sinus node 23
Root mean square of successive differences (RMSSD) 96
R-to-R intervals 86, 87, 91

Sample rate 47
SDANN statistic 97
Signal averaging 17, 115, 118
Signal processing 54, 115
    Averaging of signal 17, 115, 118
    Correlation coefficient 117, 118
    Jitter 118
    Noise detection 45, 47
    Noise monitoring 115
    Noise rejection 47, 59
    Noise removal 45
    Residual noise 119
    Signal averaging 17
    Signal-to-noise ratio (SNR) 119
    Timing errors 118
        Jitter 118
    Triggering 51, 115, 117
Signal-to-noise ratio (SNR) 119
Sinus node 23
    Arrest 25
    Arrhythmia 25
    Bradycardia 24
    Normal sinus rhythm 23
    Tachycardia 24, 33, 71
Spectral analysis, of heart rate variability
    Autoregressive 87, 101
    Box-Counting algorithm 106
    Discrete-Fourier transform (DFT) 101
    Fast-Fourier transform (FFT) 51
    Fractal (or Hausdorff) dimension 106
    Graphics, use of 91
    Grassberger-Proccacia algorithm 106
    Hyperparametric (nonparametric) DFT/FFT 101
    Nonlinear dynamic systems analysis techniques 87
    Nonparametric DFT/FFT 101
    Takens-Ellner algorithm 106
    Traditional 87, 101
Spectrotemporal mapping (STM) 133
ST segment 59, 61-69, 111, 123, 133
    Blackman-Harris function 133
    Depression of 65, 68
        Transient 68-69
        Ventricular arrhythmias and 68
    Monitoring of 59, 65
    Normal 61
    Rectangular windows function 129, 133

Sudden cardiac death (SCD) 86, 145
Sudden infant death syndrome (SIDS) 86
Supraventricular tachycardia 33, 42, 55, 71, 81, 83, 137
Tachycardia 24, 33, 83
    Infant ventricular type 79
    Junctional ectopic tachycardia (JET) 81
    Permanent junctional reciprocating tachycardia (PJRT) 81
    Supraventricular type 33, 42, 55, 71, 81, 83, 137
Tachyarrhythmia(s) 7, 75, 85
    Atrial 29
        Multifocal 28
        Paroxysmal 29
    Chaotic atrial 75
    Sinus node, in 23-26, 33, 71
Takens-Ellner algorithm 106
Threshold trigger, for heart beat 51
Time conversion factors 95
    Arithmetic mean, of heart rate 95
    Harmonic mean, of heart rate 95
Time domain analysis 121
    Bandpass filters 123
        Highpass 123
        Lowpass 123
    High-resolution ECG 121
Transesophageal 134, 141
    Pacing 134, 141
    Recording 134, 141
Transformations 47
    Amplitude-Zone-Time-Epoch-Coding (AZTEC) 47
Transient ischemia 61, 68-69
    Clinical significance 68
    Electrocardiographic features 68
        Clinical significance of 68
T wave 61, 79, 111, 143
    Monitoring of 61
    Normal 61

Vectorcardiogram (VCG) 11, 19
    Myocardial infarction 19
    Reconstruction of 19
    Standard 12-lead ECG, from 19
Vectorcardiography 11, 19
Vector magnitude waveform 123, 127
    Low amplitude signal (LAS) 127
    QRS duration 127
    QRS offset 123
    QRS onset 123
    RMS40 127
Ventricles
    Accelerated ventricular rhythm 33
    Arrhythmias originating in 33, 35
    Premature ventricular complexes (PVC) 33, 68
    Tachycardia 33, 34, 42, 111, 135, 145
    Ventricular asystole 33, 36, 42
    Ventricular fibrillation 33, 35, 41, 55, 79, 135, 143
    Ventricular flutter 33, 143
Ventricular
    Asystole 33, 36, 42
    Electrograms 7
    Fibrillation 33, 35, 41, 55, 79, 135, 143
    Flutter 33, 143
    Hypertrophy 19, 73

Wandering atrial pacemaker (WAP) 27
Wenckebach 37
    Type I second-degree AV block 37
Wolff-Parkinson-White (WPW) syndrome 81, 134, 139, 141